The American Red Cross
First Aid and Safety Handbook

About the American Red Cross

The American Red Cross is a humanitarian organization, led by volunteers, that provides relief to victims of disasters and helps people prevent, prepare for, and respond to emergencies. It does this through services that are consistent with its congressional charter and the fundamental principles of the International Red Cross Movement.

About Dr. Handal

Kathleen A. Handal, M.D., is a nationally and internationally known emergency medicine physician.

She has promoted the growth and improvement of emergency medical care for more than fifteen years, including holding leadership positions in academics and government.

As an educator, author, and lecturer, Dr. Handal has been an advocate of first aid education for everyone.

A member of the American College of Emergency Physicians, Dr. Handal attended the Medical College of Pennsylvania, is certified by the American Board of Emergency Medicine, and presently practices emergency medicine at a trauma center in Phoenix, Arizona.

Printed Exclusively for Time Inc. Home Entertainment

The American Red Cross

First Aid and Safety Handbook

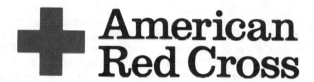

American
Red Cross

and

Kathleen A. Handal, M.D.

Foreword by Elizabeth Dole

Little, Brown and Company

Boston   New York   Toronto   London

First Edition

This book does not constitute the practice of medicine. It is not to be used instead of seeking the services of a physician, but as a guide until medical assistance is obtained.

　　The American Red Cross recommends formal first aid and CPR training for everyone. It is particularly important that CPR be learned through a certified course. Please contact your local Red Cross chapter for information on courses in your community.

　　The emergency care procedures outlined in this book reflect the standard of knowledge and accepted emergency practices in the United States at the time this book was published. We urge you, the reader, to stay informed of changes in emergency care procedures.

Library of Congress Cataloging-in-Publication Data

The American Red Cross first aid and safety handbook / [prepared by] the
　American Red Cross and Kathleen A. Handal. — 1st ed.
　　　　p.　　　cm.
　　　Includes index.
　　　ISBN 0-316-73645-7 (hc)
　　　ISBN 0-316-73646-5 (pb)
　　　1. First aid in illness and injury — Handbooks, manuals, etc.
I. Handal, Kathleen A.　II. American Red Cross.
RC86.8.A44　　1992
616.02'52 — dc20　　　　　　　　　　　　　　　　　91-24847

HC: 10　9　8　7　6　5　4
PB: 10　9　8　7　6　5　4

BP　　　

Printed in the United States of America

Contents

Part 2: First Aid   37

Part 3: Personal and Family Safety   211

Acknowledgments

Our sincere thanks to Nellie Sabin, Maura Kennedy, Don May, Lynne Filderman, Rocky Lopes, Charlotte Walhay, Jeanne Luschin, Ralph DeCesare, Ellen Denison, Jennifer Josephy, Barbara Werden, Betty Power, Lawrence Newell, Carol Robinson, Carla Brennan, Nathan Davies, Kathleen Matthews, Cyndee Archer, Robin Smith, Miley Bell, Steve Grumbacher, and John Riina for their many and varied contributions — not the least of which was patience.

Foreword

In the early part of this century, you could visit almost any American household and count on finding three books: the Bible, the works of Shakespeare, and an American Red Cross first aid textbook. People kept the Red Cross text in their home not because there were more injuries in those days, but as a kind of protective symbol. The practice was proof of the confidence Americans held in the Red Cross. It's as if our grand-parents were saying, "I trust the Red Cross because I know the Red Cross has the information I need in an emergency." Even in the days when doctors actually made house calls, it was still very important — and very American — to rely on our own resources to solve problems until pro-fessional help arrived.

What was true then is even more true today. With all the advances that have been made since those early days, no health care is more essential than knowing instantly what to do in an emergency. We all know stories of lives that have been saved by fast action on the part of friends or family members. That should be motivation enough for each of us to learn basic first aid and safety. Almost as important to the victim is the reassurance of knowing that someone close knows what to do and is doing everything that can be done. No matter how small the injury, that reassurance can be essential to recovery because it sends the tender message that someone cares.

Knowledge *is* caring. The book you hold in your hand can be a life-saver in an emergency. It is designed to give you and your family accu-rate information in the fastest possible manner when you need it most. While it's not the kind of book you read from beginning to end, please take the time to familiarize yourself with the way it works so it can help you when you need it. *The American Red Cross First Aid and Safety Handbook* is for more than just emergencies: it also contains a gold mine of information about precautions you and your family can take *today* to make your home and the lives of those you love safer and happier. Inside, there is information you need to help *prevent* emergencies from happening — always the best first aid.

The American Red Cross First Aid and Safety Handbook is not intended to replace a Red Cross training course. Red Cross health and safety courses are available in most communities and range from short, basic classes to much more sophisticated courses for emergency care professionals. Call the Red Cross chapter nearest you and find out what they offer that meets your needs. You might get so involved that you end up volunteering to provide care at a disaster or help run a blood drive or teach a first aid course or even help the Red Cross find new ways to help others. I've been a Red Cross volunteer, and it's made a wonderful difference in my life. It can enrich yours, too.

Elizabeth Dole
President
American Red Cross

Introduction: Personal Words to the Reader

As a young physician, I recall my father, John A. Handal, M.D., inscribing in my heaviest medical textbook the words "Treat always the patient, not just the disease." I've tried always to remember those words, often by spending more than the clinically necessary time with my patients.

I believe this book expands on this adage. You have a role, probably the most important one, in caring for your and others' health and safety. You are at one end of the "care chain," I and my fellow emergency physicians at the other. Common sense dictates that you and other laypersons have the greatest potential to make a difference, particularly in life-threatening emergencies.

Yes, you can make a difference. You can make an accurate report from the site of an accident so that a dispatcher can coordinate the most effective emergency response. You can care for minor emergencies and keep serious injuries from getting worse before medical help arrives. You can take steps to prevent injuries in your home, and you can be prepared to cope with disasters.

This book isn't a substitute for medical help, but a supplement to it. It's about prevention (keeping injuries from occurring) and intervention (using current and accepted methods of responding to emergencies and performing first aid).

Part 1 of this book will teach you how to think about emergencies and prepare yourself to be an effective rescuer.

Part 2 is an alphabetical listing of the major situations requiring first aid. You'll learn what first aid measures to take when an injury or illness occurs and how to recognize a life-threatening emergency. Although this book contains instructions for giving rescue breathing and CPR, it's important to get classroom training. CPR courses are available all over the nation. You'll learn more about how to recognize when CPR is needed and have a chance to gain hands-on practice in using this life-saving skill.

In Part 3, you'll find out how to minimize the chances of injury by taking steps to make your home and your activities safer. You'll also learn how to prepare for and cope with natural and man-made disasters.

Now that you have this book, use it for mock drills of emergency situations. Assemble your first aid kit, then practice and become comfortable with the first aid skills so you'll be ready in an emergency. You'll learn many simple ways to make your world safer.

The Red Cross and I share a goal: to prevent, prepare for, and cope with emergencies. Join us.

This book is dedicated to all those who know they tried to make a difference.

Kathleen A. Handal, M.D.

In an Emergency

When You Are the Rescuer

As a lay "rescuer," your role is to identify and give first aid for a life-threatening condition until medical help arrives.

By acting appropriately and quickly, you can change the outcome of many emergencies. It's nice to know you can make a difference to someone in distress — but it's also a tremendous responsibility. You'll feel more confident in the role of rescuer when you follow some common-sense rules.

Before You Act

You should consider certain aspects of giving first aid *before* you are confronted with a crisis. By thinking through these points ahead of time, you'll be able to move smoothly and effectively when your actions really count.

Be Realistic

Most people are intrigued by the idea of rescuing someone from an emergency — after all, giving emergency care can be very rewarding. We'd all like to believe that the rescuer is a hero and the grateful victim will live happily ever after.

The reality can be very different. The rescuer may find he or she can do little to help, or the victim may be uncooperative, or the situation may be extremely upsetting, or your best attempts at first aid may fail. But if you are motivated by a concern for others, you'll always have the satisfaction of knowing that you did your best to help.

What Is a Rescuer?

A rescuer is anyone who helps someone. It's you when you rush to the aid of your child when he falls off his bike, or when you give first aid at the site of a major traffic accident. In most cases, you'll be using this book for minor emergencies at home or where you work. But the principles outlined in Part 1 apply to all kinds of emergencies, from the most minor to the major.

Take the time to read it now, and it will teach you how to think about emergencies and prepare yourself to be an effective rescuer.

3

Know Yourself

Before helping someone, you need to know and understand yourself — your strengths and your limitations, both physical and emotional. How much can you push, carry, or drag? If you have physical problems — a bad back, for example — your efforts could make an emergency situation worse instead of better. If you have an excitable personality, you may worry that you'll panic in an emergency. In fact, you may find that you're stronger under pressure than you realize. Many people are, especially if they are helping a family member or friend.

To be truly effective, you need a sound understanding of yourself. If you recognize that you don't cope well with certain situations, you'll know when to turn over the rescuing to someone else. On the other hand, you may find that if you pause, take a few deep breaths, and focus on what brings you strength — for example, your concern for another person — you are able to use your knowledge and skills when they are most needed.

Remember, there is one very important step you can take in *any* emergency: calling for help.

Know the Facts

In cases where you need to perform first aid on someone outside your family, you'll want to be aware of two legal issues.

Being a Good Samaritan. You may have wondered if you can give first aid without fear of being held liable for the injuries suffered by the victim. Nearly all states have Good Samaritan laws, which are meant to encourage citizens to stop and help in an emergency. While the laws vary from state to state, most protect the lay rescuer from liability as long as he or she doesn't do anything that can be defined as grossly negligent or that shows willful misconduct — deliberately harming someone.

Know the law in your state. To find out about it, check with your police department, your public library, or a local attorney.

Obtaining Consent. Another legal issue of concern during an emergency is that of *consent*. Is the victim willing to accept your help? The victim must give his or her consent before you can administer first aid. If he or she is conscious, ask if you may help. If the victim is a minor (under 18 years old), ask the parent or guardian. If that person isn't available, the law presumes that he or she would want the child cared for in an emergency. This is called *implied consent*. If the victim is unconscious, mentally ill, emotionally disturbed, mentally retarded, or cannot think clearly because of the illness or injury, consent is also implied.

If someone refuses your help, don't argue, but don't abandon the victim either, especially if you feel the person may be confused or disoriented. Get medical help.

Be Prepared

The better prepared you are, the more likely it is that you'll be able to make a difference in a wide variety of situations. The best way to prepare for an emergency is to receive formal training in first aid and cardiopulmonary resuscitation (CPR). While this book provides instructions on when and how to perform CPR, you should carry it out only if you have been trained through a certified course. The American Red Cross offers a variety of courses in first aid and CPR. Contact your local chapter for times and locations. The hands-on practice you'll have in a class will make you feel more confident using these skills in an emergency.

Gather Your Supplies

In an emergency, it helps to have not only knowledge but also the right tools. Take the time to assemble emergency supplies before you need them, and keep them current by periodically checking them. To make a first aid kit, see A Basic First Aid Kit, page 6. Also see guidelines for emergency equipment to put in your car or truck on page 283.

An Emergency Information Chart is included in the appendixes. Make copies for your home and workplace. For your home, fill in the emergency phone numbers and other information and post the chart by your home phone. Post another in your workplace so that anyone calling for help can give, not guess, the right information in an emergency.·

Recognizing the Need to Act

To make a difference to others, learn to recognize the signs of an emergency or potential emergency. When you hear the crunch of steel and glass, you know there has been an automobile accident. Screams or calls for help are difficult to ignore. But in many emergencies, there is no dramatic call for help. A victim who is drowning, for example, or who suddenly becomes gravely ill, may not be able to tell you what is wrong or how you can help.

Train all of your senses — sight, smell, hearing, touch, even taste — to be alert to danger. Familiarize yourself with potential hazards around your home, workplace, and community, and learn as much as you can about how to handle different kinds of emergencies. When an emergency does arise, you'll know immediately that you must act — and your prompt response may save precious seconds.

A Basic First Aid Kit

Minor first aid emergencies can often be treated on the spot. You can use instructions from a knowledgeable source (for example, a physician, your local Poison Control Center, or a copy of this book) or your own experience. Having the right supplies nearby can make a difference.

A home or office first aid kit is intended mainly for minor emergencies, but it should also contain supplies that will enable you to deal with more serious injuries until the victim receives professional medical care.

First aid kits are important because they contain everything you might need in an emergency, they're portable, and they keep all of your "tools" in one place. Should an emergency occur, your first aid kit will enable you to act immediately. Your home medicine chest is not a substitute. If you have your supplies organized ahead of time, you'll save yourself both time and anxiety.

It's a good idea to familiarize yourself with the contents of your first aid kit ahead of time. You can buy a prepackaged first aid kit from most pharmacies, or you can make up your own first aid kit.

Put the first aid kit in a known and accessible place for all family members or co-workers to use — placing it near a fire extinguisher is a possibility. Don't store it in an area of extreme temperature, such as near heat or in a bathroom. Keep it on an upper shelf out of reach of children. Don't allow it to become a storage place for anything and everything related to medicine, and don't keep old medicines inside it.

To make your own kit, use a small tote bag or sturdy box big enough to be seen but small enough to carry easily. Start with a copy of this book, including a filled-out copy of the Emergency Information Chart (Appendix B) and a copy of the First Aid Kit Checklist (Appendix A). Then assemble the additional materials listed below. They can be found easily at your local pharmacy. Remember to add any special items needed by you, members of your family, or your co-workers — an allergy kit, for example.

Dressings

- Adhesive bandage strips (assorted sizes)
- Butterfly bandages
- Elastic bandage, 3 inches wide
- Hypoallergenic adhesive tape (to secure dressings in place)
- Roller bandages (a roll of stretchable gauze used to hold dressings in place)
- Sterile cotton balls
- Sterile eye patches
- Sterile gauze pads, 4 by 4 inches (individually wrapped)
- Sterile nonstick pads (to use with sterile gauze pads; combine into sterile dressings of various sizes)
- Triangular bandage (for slings or as a covering or dressing)

Instruments

- Blunt-tipped scissors (for cutting bandages or clothing)
- Tweezers (to remove splinters and other foreign objects *except* stingers from insect bites)
- Bulb syringe (to rinse eyes or wounds)

Equipment

- Cotton swabs
- Eye cup or small plastic cup
- Instant-acting chemical cold packs (for sprains, bruises, etc.)
- Paper cups (to administer fluids or use as a protective covering over a wound)
- Space blanket (for warmth)
- Thermometer (one that is easy to use)

Medication

- Activated charcoal (for poisoning emergency)
- Antiseptic wipes or antiseptic solution
- Antibiotic ointment
- Antiseptic/anesthetic spray
- Calamine/antihistamine lotion
- Sterile eye wash
- Syrup of ipecac (for use with professional medical advice during a poisoning emergency)

Miscellaneous

- Change for pay phone
- Candle and matches
- Flashlight (check batteries periodically)
- Pad and pen or pencil (check pen from time to time)
- Packet of tissues
- Soap (for cleansing wounds, scratches, cuts)
- Safety pin (for use with triangular bandage)
- Disposable latex gloves

After the immediate crisis is over, complications sometimes arise — for example, a victim may go into shock, or a wound may become infected. If you know what to watch for, you'll recognize when further action is needed.

During an Emergency

You're going to try to help a fellow human being in distress. Now what? No emergency is quite like any other, but the following guidelines will help you through any situation.

Remain Calm

Emergencies are volatile situations, and a great deal depends upon your being able to keep your wits about you. You need to think clearly, and you need to avoid making others more anxious. Emotions are contagious. A victim may not realize an injury is serious but may react to panic in the eyes or voice of a rescuer, relative, or bystander. A calm atmosphere can do wonders in preventing a situation from becoming worse.

You may have strong feelings about what has happened or is happening. You may need to tell yourself not to panic. Try at all times to focus on what you can do to help, and do so in a steady, reassuring manner. Be confident; you *will* be able to help.

Use Common Sense

Sometimes the simplest thing you can do to aid someone in distress — for example, reassuring him or her that help is on the way — is also the most helpful. Let your common sense be your guide. If you're the only rescuer, do the best you can under the circumstances. You may not always be able to change the outcome of an emergency, but give it your all and trust your instincts.

Be Resourceful

If you don't have the exact tools you need during an emergency, improvise. Use the basic first aid concepts you've learned and the materials you find at hand. You may be able to make what you need — a cup from foil, a bandage from a shirt, a splint from newspapers or pillows. Your substitute may not be perfect, but you can make it work in an emergency.

Keep Evaluating the Risks

In many emergencies, the situation changes by the minute, sometimes by the split second. In a car wreck or a home fire, for example, your own physical and emotional condition, the victim's condition, and the environment are all subject to change. As a rescuer, you need a heightened sense of awareness. Strive to sense not only the obvious, but also the subtle — for example, the victim's decreasing alertness, or the increased level of smoke. Try to respond quickly to changes. In an emergency, the unexpected can and does happen, but continuously monitoring all the risks involved will help you prevent the situation from suddenly worsening.

Do No Further Harm

This is one of the golden rules of emergency care, one with which you will become familiar as you read through this book. When giving first aid, it is possible to make an error in judgment and to do physical or emotional harm to the victim. However, this concern should never prevent you from attempting to help someone in trouble.

Don't make assumptions about the victim's physical or mental condition — he or she may be stronger or weaker than it appears at first glance. Learn as much as you can about CPR and first aid through courses and reading. Don't feel you should try something beyond your skills. Get help — often this is the best and only action for you to take, and this alone can save a life.

Chapter 2

Arriving at the Scene

The scene of an emergency can be as straightforward as a playground on which a child has fallen from a jungle gym or as complicated as the site of an industrial accident or a tornado. Only after you have quickly but carefully evaluated the circumstances will you be able to determine what steps to take.

If you're the first on the scene, or the first to assume a leadership role, use common sense to help figure out the situation. Start forming a plan of action right away. You must set priorities, starting now.

Suppose you have just arrived at the site of an emergency. As you quickly survey the scene, you need to do four things:

- Make sure the scene is safe to approach.
- If it is, determine how many people are involved.
- Try to determine what happened.
- Ask bystanders to help.

Make Sure the Scene Is Safe

First, survey the entire scene of the emergency. Is it safe, or are dangers present? For example, can you smell or see gas leaking from a wrecked car? Is it stable or likely to change? Are high winds likely to spread a now-small fire? What is the greatest danger right now? You don't want your actions to jeopardize you or the victim(s) further. Remember, your own safety is your first and most important concern. You won't be able to help anyone if you become a victim, too.

In an unsafe environment, do what you can — without endangering yourself — to make the scene secure and to prevent further accidents. Saving others from becoming victims may be a major contribution. In some cases, setting up flares or markers around an auto wreck and creating a safe area may keep others from getting hurt. If possible, ask bystanders to help keep the scene safe and to keep spectators away from the victim.

If the scene is unsafe, it may be necessary to move a victim out of the way of further harm — but *only* if his or her life is in danger. (For more about immediate rescue, see page 20.) The general rule is to move the victim *only if you absolutely have to.*

You may determine that the best thing you can do is call for help. You may not be able to reach the victim, or you may realize that you cannot evaluate the extent of the emergency on your own, or the situation may call for skills you don't have. Depending upon the circumstances, getting help may be your first priority.

Determine How Many People Are Involved

If no other rescuers are on the scene, try to quickly identify the number of victims and to assess the extent of their illnesses or injuries before you call for medical help. If there are more than three victims, don't waste time making a precise count — make a quick estimate. When you call for help, make it clear that your count is an estimate. Next, look carefully for other victims who may need your help. Remember, seriously ill or injured people may be unable to speak, moan, or cry.

As you aid the victim, reassure any family, friends, or bystanders. Remember that the other people involved are experiencing some stress, too, even if they are not ill or injured.

Try to Determine What Happened

Make no assumptions about the nature of an emergency until you have gathered as much information as possible. Ask questions at the scene. If a victim is conscious, ask him or her what happened and where he or she has been hurt. If a victim is unconscious, look around for clues that will help you discover what happened and focus on what needs to be done. You will need as much information as possible for two important reasons: first, to guide your immediate care of the victim, and second, to give it over the phone when you call for help.

Sometimes a victim's illness or injury is easy to recognize, but sometimes it isn't. Your initial evaluation is very important because it can help you avoid doing further harm to the victim. For example, you can suspect that a person lying at the bottom of a staircase has fallen and might have an injured neck or back (spine) and therefore should not be moved.

Many people with medical problems carry important information on

What to Do

- Do get help.
- Do be cautious.
- Do make sure it is safe for you to approach the victim(s).
- Do take steps to make the scene of the emergency safe — if you can do so without endangering yourself.
- Do find out as much as you can about the situation.
- Do reassure the victim and others.
- Do keep spectators away from the victim.

What Not to Do

- Do no further harm.
- Do not risk your own life or jeopardize your own safety.
- Do not panic.

a necklace, bracelet, or card. This kind of emergency medical identification can save the life of a victim who can't communicate after an accident or sudden illness.

When you call for help, the more information you can provide, the faster and more effective the medical help will be. For example, let's say the victim has swallowed a poison. If you call the Poison Control Center and can identify what the victim swallowed, the trained professional who takes your call may be able to give you instructions for first aid you can give immediately.

Sometimes special equipment and personnel are needed at the scene. The information you pass along when you call for help can bring the appropriate response more quickly.

Ask Bystanders to Help

If you're not alone, recruit bystanders to help your rescue efforts. They can help you gather the necessary information, and they may be trained in first aid and CPR. If you find yourself in a leadership role, delegate such tasks as calling for medical help and providing emotional support to the victims, their friends, and their families. Getting others to keep the area clear of onlookers or safe from traffic can contribute greatly to the victim's sense of security and to an improved rescue effort. You may end up merely discouraging spectators from staring at a victim. If so, don't belittle your role. In an emergency, not all roles are glamorous and exciting, but they *are* all important.

If possible, send someone who is familiar with the area and who knows the exact location of the emergency to watch for rescue personnel. This will help ensure that precious time is not lost as they look for the correct site.

Guidelines for Giving Emergency Care

Following certain guidelines will assist you in your role as rescuer, whatever the nature of the victim's illness or injury. By combining a step-by-step approach with your basic knowledge of the human body and how it responds to illness and injury, you may be able to make a difference to someone caught in an emergency.

Part 2 of this book gives first aid measures for specific emergencies and their related conditions. Before reviewing these, however, familiarize yourself with the following general principles of first aid.

Getting Started

You have already arrived at the emergency and made sure the scene is safe. You have quickly identified the victim(s), determined what happened, and asked bystanders to help you. What happens next?

Your initial response during these early moments of an emergency is critical. As you evaluate the circumstances and injuries and figure out what to do next, it will help to think in terms of A-I-D:

> **A**   Ask for help
> **I**   Intervene
> **D**   Do no further harm

These steps will guide you as you develop your plan of action.

Ask for Help

In a crisis, time is of the essence. The more quickly you recognize an emergency, and the faster you call for medical assistance, the sooner the victim will get help. Immediate care can greatly affect the outcome of an emergency.

What to Do

- Do obtain consent, when possible.
- Do think the worst. It's best to administer first aid for the gravest possibility.
- Do call or send for help.
- Do remember to identify yourself to the victim.
- Do provide emotional support.
- Do respect the victim's modesty and physical privacy.
- Do be as calm and as direct as possible.
- Do care for the most serious injuries first.
- Do assist the victim with his or her prescription medication.

What Not to Do

- Do no further harm.
- Do not leave the victim alone except to get help.
- Do not assume that the victim's obvious injuries are the only ones.
- Do not deny a victim's physical or emotional coping limitations.
- Do not make any unrealistic promises.
- Do not trust the judgment of a confused victim.
- Do not require the victim to make decisions.

The next chapter, Getting Medical Help, will tell you more about whom to call for expert medical advice and what to expect after you have placed a call for help.

Intervene

To "intervene" means to do something for the victim that will help achieve a positive outcome to an emergency. Sometimes getting medical help will be all you can do, and this alone may save a life. In other situations, however, you may become actively involved in the victim's initial care by giving first aid. Let the Golden Rules of Emergency Care (see box) guide your efforts.

Do No Further Harm

Once you have begun first aid, you want to be certain you don't do anything that might cause the victim's condition to worsen. Certain actions should always be avoided. By keeping them in mind, you will be able to avoid adding to or worsening the victim's illness or injuries.

How to Do No Further Harm

The following rules will help ensure that you do no further harm as you administer first aid to someone.

1. **Don't block an unconscious victim's airway (the passage that allows the person to breathe).** An unconscious victim or a victim who is having difficulty breathing may choke or suffocate if his or her airway is not protected. With that in mind:

    - *Never lay an unconscious victim flat on his or her back or face* (except to begin CPR).
    - *Never place a pillow under the head of an unconscious victim.*
    - *Never put anything, including liquids, into an unconscious victim's mouth.*

2. **Don't use force.** Avoid any first aid procedure that requires the use of force (except CPR chest compressions and abdominal thrusts for choking). With that in mind:

    - *Never forcefully test a victim for responsiveness* (for example, do not shake the victim).
    - *Never force an unconscious victim's jaws apart.*
    - *Never try to keep a convulsing victim's limbs from moving.*
    - *Never force a victim to vomit* by sticking anything, including your fingers, down his or her throat.

- *Never continue a first aid measure if it causes the victim pain.*
- *Never force any part of the body* as you administer a first aid technique.
- *Never remove an impaled object from the body.*

3. **Never move anyone who could possibly have injured his or her neck or back (spine)** unless there is urgent danger. Movement to the neck or back may cause spinal injury, which can lead to paralysis. As a general rule, don't move *any* victim unless the scene is unsafe.

4. **Never move an injured body part without supporting the injured area**. Moving an injured body part without supporting it not only increases the victim's pain but also can damage blood vessels and nerves around broken bones.

How to Approach Someone Who Is Ill or Injured

If the victim is conscious, obtain his or her consent before beginning first aid. If you don't know the person, introduce yourself, using your full name, and ask if you can help. If you have taken a first aid course, say so. Even if the victim is unconscious, friends, family, or co-workers present need to know who you are and what your intentions are as you approach him or her.

As you give first aid, it's important to continuously explain your intentions and actions and how you are going to help the victim. Keep reassuring the person, although you should be careful not to make unrealistic promises.

While the first aid depends on the situation, you'll always begin by performing a complete evaluation of the victim's condition.

How to Evaluate the Victim's Condition

When you administer first aid, your first priority is to care for any life-threatening conditions. The first things to do when you approach someone who has become ill or injured are to see if the person is conscious and to check his or her vital body functions. This is basic to all the first aid procedures given in Part 2.

All true life-or-death conditions center on the proper functioning of the heart and lungs (the respiratory and circulatory systems). In order for the body to work properly, the heart must keep pumping oxygenated blood from the lungs to the brain. If the victim is not breathing, if his or her heart has stopped, or if he or she is bleeding severely, immediate action is required.

To find out if the respiratory and circulatory systems are working, you must check the ABCs — Airway, Breathing, and Circulation.

Airway. The passage through which a person breathes, the airway, must be clear so he or she can breathe.

Breathing. A person must breathe to survive.

Circulation. A person must have adequate circulation. That means that he or she must have a pulse. It also means that he or she must not be bleeding severely.

After you have tested the victim for consciousness (see next section), check his or her ABCs and continue monitoring them until medical help arrives.

If the victim is not breathing, you will need to begin *rescue breathing* (also known as mouth-to-mouth resuscitation) at once. If the victim has no circulation because his or her heart has stopped beating, you'll need to begin *chest compressions* immediately. When performed together, these techniques are known as cardiopulmonary resuscitation, or CPR. (CPR procedures for infants and young children vary slightly from the techniques used on adults. All of these are described in detail under **Cardiopulmonary Arrest** on page 89.) The victim's circulation is also in danger if there is heavy bleeding. You will have to take steps to control the bleeding (page 62).

In all emergencies, maintaining or restoring the victim's ABCs — airway, breathing, and circulation — is the top priority. CPR is a way of manually attempting to restore a victim's vital body functions. *CPR should be learned through a certified course* (contact your Red Cross chapter for information). Getting formal training in CPR is the best way to prepare yourself for giving first aid to someone whose ABCs are not present.

Checking for Consciousness

Since an unconscious person requires special treatment, you must immediately determine whether or not the victim is conscious. Tap him or her gently and ask, "Are you OK?" If the victim is conscious and alert, it will be easier for you to find out what happened and determine what needs to be done. If the victim is unconscious and you did not witness his or her collapse, the first aid measures you take will depend upon how much you can discover about the illness or injury.

If the Victim Is Conscious

If you have established that the victim is conscious and breathing normally, you won't need to start rescue breathing. Continue your evaluation by checking the victim's circulation — that is, by checking his or her pulse and looking for any evidence of severe bleeding. If necessary, take steps to control heavy bleeding by administering first aid for bleeding. (See **Bleeding** on page 62.)

Continue to check the victim's ABCs. If the victim's illness or injury is severe, his or her condition may deteriorate and rescue breathing or CPR may become necessary. If the victim's pulse weakens, slows, or stops completely, or if the victim loses consciousness, this can signal grave danger. Be prepared to begin CPR while you wait for medical help.

If the Victim Is Unconscious

To evaluate an unconscious victim's ABCs, follow the step-by-step sequence given in the following emergency action plan. The detailed techniques for each step of this plan are discussed in greater depth in other sections of this book, but the essential steps are as follows:

1. **Check for neck or back injury**. *If you suspect a spinal injury*, leave the victim in the position found while you try to evaluate his or her ABCs. If the ABCs do not seem to be present and *you do not suspect a spinal injury*, turn the victim onto his or her back, rolling the body as a unit and supporting the head and neck as best you can.

2. **If you do not suspect a spinal injury,** open the victim's airway by tilting his or her head back and lifting up his or her chin (Figure 1). (The head-tilt/chin-lift method is described in more detail under **Cardiopulmonary Arrest** on page 89.) **If you do suspect a spinal injury**, open the airway with a chin lift. Do not use the head tilt.

3. **Look, listen, and feel for breathing**. Look to see if the chest is rising and falling, listen for breathing, and feel for escaping air against your cheek (Figure 2). Chest movement alone does not mean that the victim is breathing.

    If the victim is breathing, continue your evaluation by checking his or her circulation. (See Step 4.)

    If the victim is not breathing, begin rescue breathing by giving 2 full breaths (Figure 3). (Rescue breathing is described in detail under **Cardiopulmonary Arrest** on page 89.) Then check the victim's circulation. (See Step 4.)

    If you attempt rescue breathing but the chest does not rise and fall and you cannot feel escaping air, tilt the victim's head farther back and attempt 2 more breaths.

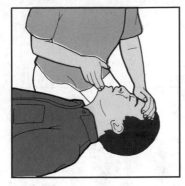
Figure 1
Head tilt/chin lift

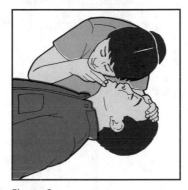
Figure 2
Look, listen, and feel for breathing

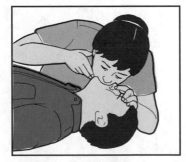
Figure 3
Begin rescue breathing

If the victim's chest still does not rise, his or her airway is obstructed. Begin first aid for an unconscious victim who is choking. (See **Choking** on page 108.)

If the victim begins to breathe again, move to Step 4.

4. **Check the victim's circulation**. Both a pulse and a sufficient amount of blood within the body are needed for adequate circulation.

   Check the victim's pulse by feeling his or her carotid artery. Place your fingers in the groove between the victim's voice box and the muscle of his or her neck (Figure 4). Feel for a pulse for 5 to 10 seconds. (For an infant, check the brachial pulse in the arm — see page 95.)

   Look for any evidence of heavy bleeding. If necessary, take steps to control any heavy bleeding. (See **Bleeding** on page 62.)

5. How you care for the victim from this point depends upon the condition of his or her ABCs.

   If the victim has no pulse and is not breathing, begin CPR. (See **Cardiopulmonary Arrest** on page 89.)

   If the victim has a pulse but is not breathing, continue to perform rescue breathing only.

   If the victim has a pulse and is breathing, continue to closely monitor his or her ABCs as you evaluate the victim's condition and give first aid for the illness or injuries.

   Call the Emergency Medical Services (EMS) system for help if you have not done so already.

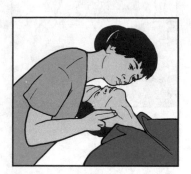

Figure 4
Check the victim's pulse on the side of the neck

Moving the Victim

The best position for a victim depends on what kind of illness or injuries he or she has. In general, the best position for an injured or ill person is lying down flat, since this improves the body's circulation and protects the airway. Helping to place the victim in an appropriate position can ease his or her discomfort and help prevent complications. However, if you're not sure about the correct position in which to put a victim with a given injury, keep him or her lying as found.

Do not change a victim's position until you have made sure no neck or back injury has occurred. If anything about the scene leads you to believe that the victim has fallen or has suffered any trauma (direct bodily harm from forces outside the body) to the head or face, wait for professional help before moving him or her, since serious neck injury can be

The Emergency Action Plan

This chart shows the steps you should follow when approaching someone who is ill or injured. If the victim's condition is serious or deteriorating, focus your attention on the ABCs — airway, breathing, and circulation — and **call the Emergency Medical Services (EMS) system as soon as possible**.

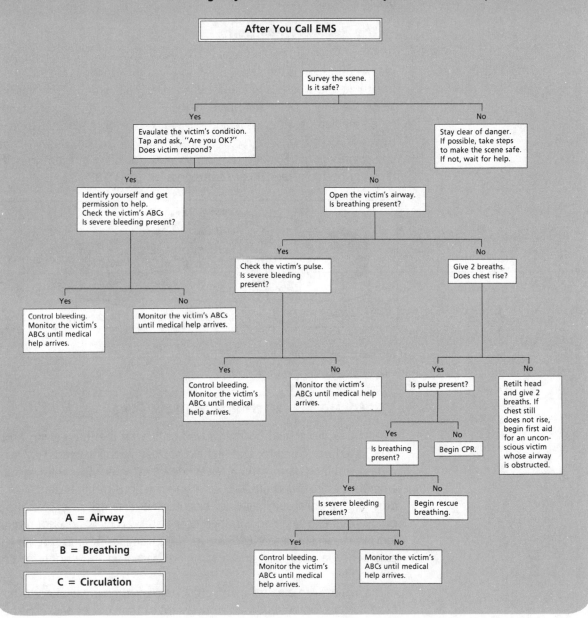

After You Call EMS

Survey the scene. Is it safe?

Yes → Evaulate the victim's condition. Tap and ask, "Are you OK?" Does victim respond?

No → Stay clear of danger. If possible, take steps to make the scene safe. If not, wait for help.

Evaulate the victim's condition:

Yes → Identify yourself and get permission to help. Check the victim's ABCs Is severe bleeding present?

No → Open the victim's airway. Is breathing present?

Is severe bleeding present?

Yes → Control bleeding. Monitor the victim's ABCs until medical help arrives.

No → Monitor the victim's ABCs until medical help arrives.

Open the victim's airway. Is breathing present?

Yes → Check the victim's pulse. Is severe bleeding present?

No → Give 2 breaths. Does chest rise?

Check the victim's pulse. Is severe bleeding present?

Yes → Control bleeding. Monitor the victim's ABCs until medical help arrives.

No → Monitor the victim's ABCs until medical help arrives.

Give 2 breaths. Does chest rise?

Yes → Is pulse present?

No → Retilt head and give 2 breaths. If chest still does not rise, begin first aid for an unconscious victim whose airway is obstructed.

Is pulse present?

Yes → Is breathing present?

No → Begin CPR.

Is breathing present?

Yes → Is severe bleeding present?

No → Begin rescue breathing.

Is severe bleeding present?

Yes → Control bleeding. Monitor the victim's ABCs until medical help arrives.

No → Monitor the victim's ABCs until medical help arrives.

A = Airway

B = Breathing

C = Circulation

present in these situations. A victim with a neck or back injury who is moved by someone without the correct training and equipment could be paralyzed. Unless there is *urgent* danger, wait for a trained rescue crew. You should know that cars involved in a wreck rarely catch fire.

If the scene is unsafe and you *must* move the victim, there are special techniques you can use. (See Immediate Rescue from an Unsafe Area below.)

The Recovery Position

So long as you have no reason to suspect a neck or back injury, the recovery position is the safest position for an unconscious victim who is breathing and who has not suffered any trauma (Figure 5). This position keeps the airway open and prevents the victim from inhaling any fluids; he or she can breathe easily and will not choke on his or her tongue. However, *do not use the recovery position if you suspect the victim has any spinal injury*. (For information on how to move a victim into the recovery position, see **Unconsciousness** on page 182.)

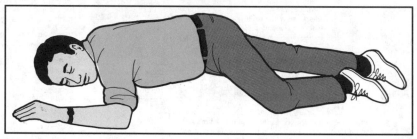

Figure 5
The recovery position

Immediate Rescue from an Unsafe Area

Ideally, a victim should not be moved until after life-threatening problems have been cared for and first aid has been administered. However, certain situations are in themselves life-threatening. Examples include emergencies involving fire, lack of oxygen, serious traffic hazard, risk of drowning, a collapsing building, electrical hazard, risk of explosion, or exposure to extreme bad weather. Many auto accidents do *not* require moving the victim before EMS arrives. In a true life- or limb-threatening emergency, all decisions and actions are based on the priority of preserving life.

If a victim with a spinal injury must be moved, you will need to take extreme care. Do not allow any movement of the neck or back. It is best to transport the victim on a board or other rigid surface. (See How to Move a Victim with a Suspected Spinal Injury on page 178.)

Following are some techniques you can use to move a victim from an unsafe area.

Immediate Rescue with One Rescuer

If the scene is unsafe and you must move a victim by yourself before professional help arrives, you can use the *clothes drag technique* on page 178. This technique requires no special equipment, supports the victim's head and neck, and can be done even if you are alone. This technique is appropriate if, owing to a dangerous environment, you are forced to move a victim who has a spinal injury; it is discussed in detail under **Spinal Injury** (see page 175). If the victim is large, you can use the *foot drag technique* as long as the surface over which the victim is dragged is not rough or bumpy. Hold the victim's ankles as you pull the person to safety. *Do not use the foot drag technique if you suspect spinal injury.*

Immediate Rescue with Two Rescuers

If the scene is unsafe and there is only one other person on hand who can help you move the victim, use the *two-handed seat carry* (Figure 6). Use this technique only if the victim has no serious injuries and is able to cooperate with the rescuers. *Never use this technique if the victim may have injured his or her spine.*

Immediate Rescue with Three Rescuers

If the scene is unsafe and several bystanders are available to assist you in moving the victim, use the *three-person hammock carry* (Figure 7).

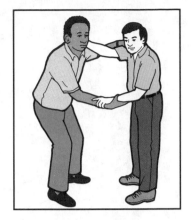

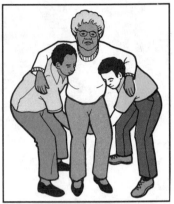

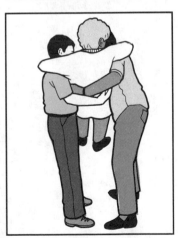

Figure 6
The two-handed seat carry

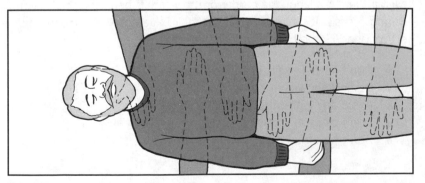

Figure 7
The three-person hammock carry

Make sure the victim's head, neck, back, arms, buttocks, thighs, and knees are supported, and see that these remain in a straight line. Move toward help and only the shortest distance to safety, being careful to keep all injured body parts from twisting, bending, or shaking. If a limb is obviously broken and enough rescuers are available, have one rescuer place one hand above the injured area and one just below, keeping the bone from twisting or bending while the victim is moved. The rest of the helpers move the victim, keeping all of his or her body parts in a straight line.

Care for the Person, Not Just the Emergency

Perhaps the most important thing to remember when helping an injured or ill person is that you are caring for a fellow human being. You're not just treating a cut, a broken leg, or a heart attack; you're caring for a person who has suffered a sudden injury or illness and who may be under emotional stress. He or she may be in pain, afraid, or disoriented. If others are watching, the victim may be self-conscious as well.

Just as every accident and every emergency is different, so is each victim's ability to withstand pain or injury. The effect that a sudden illness or injury has on an individual varies greatly and depends in part on the person's physical or emotional state and the severity of the emergency.

Although each individual's response to illness or injury is unique, certain reactions are very common. Pain can make a victim feel anxious, irritable, or angry. Other common responses include depression, regression, denial, resentment, and confusion. Even calm, sensible people may be dramatically changed by a crisis, acting immature or aggressive. You can gain a great deal of information by reading the victim's body language, making eye contact, and noting his or her expressions.

Never assume that it's impossible to communicate with any victim, even if there is a language barrier or the victim is behaving unpleasantly. During a crisis, it's especially important to keep the lines of communication open. Some helpful guidelines:

- Don't let the victim make you angry.
- Respect the victim's privacy.
- Avoid any kind of excitement.
- Don't threaten the victim.
- Don't be afraid of silence.

Emergencies Involving Children

Children, too, are individuals. They have a strong sense of intuition and can sense when you are frightened or unsure. If you are relaxed, children tend to be relaxed around you. If you are panicky, children panic, too. When caring for a child who is ill or injured, try to keep your own anxiety under control, and remember that your behavior — conscious or unconscious — will affect how the child reacts to the emergency.

When speaking to a child, be reassuring and position yourself at the child's height, making eye contact. Some gentle physical contact while talking, such as resting your fingers on the child's arm lightly, is reassuring; if the child does not know you, this also helps reduce his or her fear of a stranger. Explain to the child that you know he or she is in pain but that help is on the way. Don't describe the degree of pain or the time it will take for help to arrive. Explain all your movements toward the child before you make them. As you give first aid, show the child any equipment or dressings you will be using before you use them.

Emergencies Involving Older People

When helping an older person, it's important to remember that you are dealing with a long-lived person who has had ample opportunity to become very much an individual, set in his or her own ways. Physical and emotional changes can be extremely upsetting and difficult to adjust to. When offering to help an older victim, acknowledge the disruptive nature of the emergency and be reassuring.

Ordinarily it is a good idea to avoid asking the victim to make decisions. With an older victim, however, it can be helpful to give the person as much control as possible over decisions about his or her circumstances. Don't assume that an older victim is hard of hearing and shout when speaking to him or her. Remember, too, that as we get older, we tend to speak more slowly and spend more time on words, thoughts, and conversations — not necessarily because our minds have gotten slower, but because we have learned the importance of careful verbal communication.

Emergencies Involving Victims of Crime

If you think a crime has occurred, be sure the scene is safe before attempting to help, especially if you're the first person on the scene. Tell the victim your name and make it clear that you want to help; the victim may be disoriented and frightened and may believe the ordeal is not yet over.

It's always important not to judge a victim, and this is especially true of a victim of a crime. Keep in mind that the way you treat and care for the victim in the moments after a crime can make a difference not only in his or her immediate emotional state but also in long-term recovery.

As you may imagine, someone who has been assaulted is likely to have a very emotional reaction. The victim may react with rage, hysteria, or even disbelief. The emotional emergency may be even greater than any visible physical injury. One of your top priorities is to make sure that the person isn't further traumatized by your assistance. Privacy, comfort, and dignity are essential in considering first aid to the victim of any crime, especially a rape.

Stay with the victim until police arrive. During that time, don't touch or move anything — you could destroy evidence that could be needed to prosecute the assailant.

If the Victim Dies

Occasionally, first aid and resuscitation efforts are unsuccessful — even when trained emergency personnel have administered life support. Victims are not usually pronounced dead at the scene of an emergency; they are taken to a hospital before this determination is made. However, if you're present when someone is pronounced dead, family, friends, and the others involved in the emergency may need your attention and emotional support.

If you have been involved in an unsuccessful attempt at resuscitation, don't allow this failure to shake your conviction that you can make a difference in an emergency. Try to remember that death may occur despite the very best efforts of everyone involved. We are limited in our ability to preserve life, and recognizing this is important for both the rescuer and the victim's loved ones. Even science as we know it today can't explain why a certain injury will kill one victim but not the next, and why, in some cases, death is inevitable.

As a rescuer, be aware that the same idealism that motivates you to help others also can give you unrealistic expectations. We all hope every victim will recover completely, but there are no guarantees. Even trained professionals can't always save a life. If death does occur, try to accept it and deal with it as best you can. Grieving is natural, healthy, and constructive, especially if you knew the victim; condemning yourself for the death of the victim is not.

Health Precautions and Guidelines for the Rescuer

You may be wondering if you can safely give first aid from the stand-point of your own present and future health. The answer is a guarded "yes." If you keep certain health guidelines in mind, you will be able to minimize your own health risks as you help someone else.

Physical Strain

Some health risks associated with administering first aid are related to dangers within the environment — for example, a burning building — and the limitations of your own body. As a rescuer, if you find that you are pushing yourself beyond your abilities, heed the warnings of your body. Don't expect more of yourself than you can deliver. If you have a back condition, for example, don't try to lift or drag a victim alone or without enough help. Remember, you don't want to become an additional victim.

Disease

The spread of AIDS (acquired immunodeficiency syndrome) has raised concerns about the risks of transmitting disease when giving first aid. While these fears are certainly understandable, you should know that the risk of giving or getting HIV (the virus that causes AIDS) or other serious diseases when giving first aid is very small.

Disease transmission works two ways: the rescuer can infect the victim, or the victim can infect the rescuer. If you know or suspect you have a disease or infection, you must take protective measures when you administer first aid. If you're using your first aid knowledge and skills to help someone you know well — a family member, friend, or co-worker — you will probably have some idea of that person's health status. But because there is no sure way to know whether someone is healthy, you should always adopt practices that discourage the spread of disease when you give first aid.

Blood-borne diseases and viruses, such as hepatitis and HIV, are spread through direct contact of the blood of an infected person with blood of a noninfected person through open cuts or sores on the skin or in the mouth or eyes. Unbroken skin is the best protection. To reduce contact with blood when you are trying to control bleeding, use a barrier — gloves, several dressings, plastic wrap — between you and the victim's blood whenever possible. Try to avoid direct contact with other body fluids, such as saliva, vomit, feces, and urine. And try to avoid touching surfaces or objects that have been contaminated with the blood or body fluids. Always wash your hands immediately after giving first aid, even if you wore gloves. If, despite your efforts, you did come in contact with the victim's body fluids, talk to your personal physician immediately.

Air-borne diseases such as colds and flu are spread when sneezing and coughing spray germs through the air. They can be spread through casual contact as easily as through first aid. To avoid transmitting or catching such diseases, wash your hands carefully before and after caring for a victim, even if you wore gloves.

You can be prepared by keeping antiseptic wipes and waterless soap in your first aid kit, in case soap and water aren't available.

Rescue breathing brings you into contact with the victim's saliva. This worries some people, but in fact there is only a theoretical risk of HIV infection through saliva. If you are in a situation in which you might frequently be called upon to give first aid that might require rescue breathing, you should consider taking an advanced CPR course that will train you in the use of a resuscitation mask. Using a resuscitation mask allows you to give rescue breathing without making mouth-to-mouth contact.

As a rescuer, you should be guided by your own ethical values as well as your knowledge of the risks that may be present in each situation.

Getting Medical Help

There is more than one way to get medical help, so you should familiarize yourself with the possibilities in your area. When you're unsure about what to do or are overwhelmed by the victim's sudden or worsening illness or injury, seek immediate advice from an expert. Depending upon the kind of emergency, you can call the victim's physician, the Emergency Medical Services (EMS) system, or your local Poison Control Center. It may be obvious that the victim needs to go to an emergency facility at once. Even if you believe that you can provide the needed first aid and transport the victim to the emergency facility yourself, it's a good idea to call for medical advice first.

The greatest good you can do in some situations is simply to get help. Even if the "only" action you take is to call Emergency Medical Services (EMS), you could be saving a life, and the way in which you make the call could save precious minutes.

In some emergencies, you'll have enough time to call for specific medical advice before administering first aid. But in some situations, you'll need to attend to the victim first. For example, if the victim has stopped breathing, your first priority will be to begin rescue breathing. If the victim is being electrocuted, your first step will be to turn off the current. If the victim's heart has stopped, starting cardiopulmonary resuscitation (CPR) will be the first priority.

If you are alone or isolated, you should, if possible, call for help before acting alone. Notify someone of the emergency and what measures you are taking. For example, don't go into a burning building after hearing screams if you are alone and help has not been called.

If more than one rescuer is on the scene, send a capable bystander to get help while you attend to the victim. If possible, send two people to make the call to ensure it is made accurately. Don't assume that a child can't call for help.

What happens after you call for help? That depends upon whom you have called and the nature and severity of the emergency. Most emergencies can be handled in one of the following ways:

- If EMS has been dispatched, the patient may be taken to the emergency department of the nearest hospital, or to another hospital that is specially equipped to care for this specific emergency.
- You may be advised to take the victim to the emergency department of the nearest hospital or to another emergency facility.
- You may be advised to call the victim's physician or take the victim to a physician's office.
- With the medical advice you receive over the telephone, you may be able to administer first aid on the spot. Follow-up care may or may not be necessary.

Each year more than 85 million people in the United States are treated in emergency facilities. The odds are good that you'll someday go to an emergency facility, either while accompanying a victim or as a victim yourself. Knowing in advance what to do and what you can expect will ease the stress during the medical emergency.

Activating the Emergency Medical Services (EMS) System

Call EMS if you suspect the situation is life- or limb-threatening or if the victim has suffered injuries that prevent him or her from being easily moved. (See Whom Should You Call? opposite.)

What Is EMS?

The Emergency Medical Services (EMS) system provides rapid, coordinated medical assistance in an emergency, including telephone advice, trained ambulance personnel, and equipment to stabilize and transport a victim to an emergency facility. As a result of federal legislation, a resource for EMS should be available in your area.

You should be aware that local emergency medical response capabilities are not all the same. Federal and state statutes address EMS standards, including such issues as training, operations, and even the recertification of ambulances and emergency medical technicians. However, states are not required to develop Emergency Medical Services systems to any specified or standardized level of care. In many areas, the fire or police departments provide EMS. In the greater part of the United

Whom Should You Call?

Making the right first phone call in an emergency can save precious moments, but sometimes you may not know where to turn. Here are some guidelines to help you decide.

When to Call the Emergency Medical Services (EMS) System
If the victim:

- Is not breathing and/or has no pulse
- Is having extreme difficulty breathing
- Is having convulsions or seizures
- Is unconscious
- Is showing signs of shock
- Has a serious head injury
- Has injured his or her neck or back or may have a spinal injury
- Has a possible broken bone in a weight-bearing limb or a serious fracture elsewhere
- Is passing or vomiting large amounts of blood or experiencing severe bleeding elsewhere
- Is ill or injured and cannot be easily moved
- Has a life- or limb-threatening injury or illness

  Call EMS if you are dealing with any serious medical problem.

When to Call Your Local Poison Control Center

- If you know or suspect someone has been exposed to poison, either by mouth, breathing, or skin contact

When to Call the Victim's Physician
If the victim:

- Shows signs of decreasing alertness
- Has severe diarrhea and/or vomiting
- Has a persistent high fever or a sudden rise in temperature
- Is in great pain or is suffering from pain that does not go away
- Is dehydrated (has not passed urine for 10 hours)

  And, if possible, call the victim's physician after you have called EMS, especially if the victim is dangerously ill or seriously injured.

States, EMS systems are supported by volunteer workers. Learn about and support your local EMS.

What Is an Emergency Medical Technician (EMT)?

An emergency medical technician (EMT) is a certified professional with the specific knowledge and skills needed to provide prehospital emergency care. EMTs are trained to different levels of expertise for responding with equipment and vehicles to life- or limb-threatening emergencies. Physicians supervise their education and delivery of care. Commonly, there are three levels of training for EMTs. The basic EMT can perform basic life-support procedures, including checking vital signs, performing CPR, administering oxygen, defibrillation of the heart, and applying bandages and splints. The intermediate EMT can initiate limited advanced life-support procedures under a physician's supervision; he or she can, among other things, start intravenous fluids, administer some medications, and apply defibrillators to electrically stimulate hearts. The advanced EMT is known as a paramedic. Paramedics can perform more sophisticated advanced life-support procedures and may initiate certain lifesaving procedures without a direct verbal order from a physician.

An emergency response team includes different levels of medical technicians. The same type of team is not sent to every emergency, nor are paramedics automatically sent to every emergency. Most EMS systems can provide both basic life-support service and advanced life-support service, but exactly who is dispatched to a given emergency depends upon the nature of the emergency and the resources of your local EMS system.

What's the Correct Phone Number?

It's important to become familiar with the emergency medical resources in your community and to develop a plan just in case an emergency should occur. First, you need to know how to activate EMS in your community or in the place you are visiting. The correct phone number is your link to rapid emergency medical care. In some communities, you can use the same number to reach fire, police, or EMS.

You've probably heard that you can dial 911 in an emergency and get help. In more than 50 percent of the nation, this is true — by dialing 911 you can activate an emergency medical response, the police, or fire assistance; the operator will forward your call to the appropriate agency. (You can dial 911 from pay phones in many parts of the country without inserting a coin.)

In certain communities, however, there is no 911 emergency telephone system. Be sure you find out in advance the phone number you must use to get emergency assistance. If you don't know the correct number, dial "0" and the operator will connect you to EMS.

Teach your children or grandchildren how to call EMS for help. Also teach them their phone number and their address so EMS can locate their home. Children have saved lives by summoning EMS and have even taken and followed first aid instructions from EMS dispatchers over the phone with successful results.

When Should You Call EMS?

Throughout this book, the EMS logo is used to highlight situations and points at which you should call EMS. As you read on, you'll familiarize yourself with these kinds of critical emergencies, and common sense will also be your guide. If you are in doubt about whether to phone EMS, however, go ahead and call. After gathering the necessary information from you, the EMS dispatcher will make decisions concerning dispatching EMS personnel to the scene. The EMS dispatcher can also tell you what to do during the precious minutes between your call for help and the arrival of EMS personnel.

What Happens When You Call EMS?

You activate EMS by dialing the local EMS number. When you explain that there is a medical emergency, you will be connected to an EMS dispatcher who will ask you questions. Be prepared to tell the dispatcher:

- What happened (the nature of the emergency)
- Where the emergency is, including landmarks, cross streets, the name of the building, the floor, and the apartment or room number
- The telephone number from which you are calling
- Your name
- How many people need help
- Condition of the victim(s)
- What help is being given to the victim(s)

Be sure to wait until the dispatcher has no more questions. *Do not* hang up first; let the person you call hang up first.

The dispatcher may give advice to you, the rescuer, as the EMS personnel and ambulance are being dispatched. Listen carefully. If you have any questions, ask them. Dispatchers are invaluable at instructing you how to help a victim, and they will stay on the phone and advise you while you administer first aid.

It may feel like an eternity until EMS arrives. If possible, send someone out to watch for EMS and direct rescue personnel to the scene. Usually at least two EMS professionals will arrive with equipment in a transport vehicle. Sometimes, especially in rural areas, a helicopter may arrive and an area may need to be secured for a safe landing. (These "air ambulances" are rapidly becoming more widespread.)

EMS personnel must follow certain procedures and orders in particular emergencies. These include instructions regarding medical care and the need to contact the supervising physician at the base hospital.

Your cooperation with the EMS system is the best thing for the patient. You may offer to add another set of hands to the team. Even if your only contribution is to keep the area clear as the EMS personnel care for and prepare to transport the patient, this is a vital role.

Since not all emergency facilities are equipped and staffed to the same level, each EMS system evaluates the capabilities of area emergency facilities before selecting them to receive patients. Your local EMS personnel will know where to take emergency patients with particular illnesses or injuries. If you or the victim prefers a particular emergency facility, EMS personnel may or may not be able to accommodate you. Where the victim will be taken depends upon his or her preference, past medical problems, private physician arrangements, and most important, present medical condition, as well as the capabilities of the emergency facilities in the area. If a particular emergency facility is already overcrowded, that too will affect this decision. EMS personnel can involve a physician in the destination decision by way of radio communication.

Depending upon the circumstances, the patient may be taken to one of the following:

- *The emergency department of the nearest hospital.* An emergency department is an emergency facility within a hospital. Your nearest hospital's emergency department may be able to fully handle the emergency. Sometimes a patient receives stabilizing care at the nearest hospital before being transferred elsewhere for ongoing care.
- *A hospital designated for this kind of emergency.* If the situation allows, the patient may be taken directly to the emergency department of a hospital with special treatment centers (for example, a burn center, trauma center, etc.).
- *A freestanding emergency facility,* such as an "urgent care center" or "emergicenter." These nonhospital facilities are capable of taking care of minor emergencies and urgent situations, but they are not designed to handle ambulance patients with life- or limb-threatening emergencies. After a critical patient is stabilized at a nonhospital emergency facility, he or she will be transferred for admission to a hospital for further care.

Calling the Poison Control Center

Call your regional Poison Control Center for expert information and advice regarding possible poisoning accidents or emergencies. The Poison Control Center is staffed by specially trained experts. Most areas of the United States have centers open twenty-four hours a day. They have information on hand about every possible poisonous and nonpoisonous substance, and in a poisoning emergency can give you first aid instructions over the phone. (Check the front of your local phone book for the number of your Poison Control Center.)

Most poisoning emergencies can be prevented by taking common-sense precautions. (See How to Poison-Proof Your Home on page 217.) Your Poison Control Center may have literature available that will help you prevent poisoning accidents. And since they are regional, Poison Control Centers are familiar with the poisonous substances (including plants) found in your area.

Calling the Victim's Physician

If you're uncertain about the nature of the emergency or the urgency of a medical condition, try to call the victim's physician first. He or she knows the victim, has treated him or her in the past, and may be best able to assist you. Often a conversation with the victim's physician, and his or her guidance over the phone, will save you from making an inappropriate call to EMS or an unnecessary visit to an emergency facility. But if the situation is urgent, the physician may advise you to call EMS and may become personally involved in the victim's subsequent care.

Don't assume that because it is a weekend or after hours, the victim's physician will be unavailable. The physician's answering service can locate him or her or can contact the physician covering the practice.

It's important to get professional help in evaluating an injury or illness, for it may be difficult for you, a lay rescuer, to judge the severity of an emergency. Some injuries can look worse than they are — for example, even a relatively minor cut to the scalp can bleed profusely. Other injuries may be more serious than they appear — for example, a fall from a bicycle may leave an obvious skinned knee and perhaps also a concussion.

When you call the victim's physician, remain calm. If time permits, write down your questions as well as his or her answers. Repeat the physician's instructions aloud to make sure you understand them correctly. If someone is with you, this also gives that person a chance to hear the instructions.

If the victim's physician has been notified, he or she may meet you at the emergency department. If you aren't able to reach the victim's physician before you get to the hospital, you can ask the emergency physician to make the call. In the rapid pace of an EMS response, the victim's physician is often not contacted until the victim is in the emergency department receiving care. Whether or not the emergency department physician contacts the victim's physician depends upon the victim's condition, the victim's personal request, and the private physician's preferences. Often a private physician can supply information about a patient's medical history that will help the emergency physician.

The Hospital Emergency Department

Not all hospitals participate in EMS systems. The emergency departments that participate in *most* EMS systems are required to meet a minimum level of staffing and equipment and must be available to receive emergency patients twenty-four hours a day, seven days a week.

Planning Ahead

Your EMS system or physician can help you locate the nearest emergency department. If you have more than one hospital to choose from, investigate which one is best able to meet your emergency needs. Ask your physician for a recommendation, ask your friends and neighbors about their experiences, and talk to your local EMS professionals.

Visit the emergency department in your area and familiarize yourself with its exact location and layout. Take the time to figure out the fastest route to the emergency department, both from your home and from your workplace. Find the entrance you would use in an emergency if you were to arrive by private car. Locate the parking lot, pay telephones, and bathrooms. You'll feel a bit more at home if you must return under different circumstances. It may be a good idea to take your children along for an informal look around; this will reduce their fear if they return in an emergency.

Don't be afraid to approach one of the staff with your questions. Since all emergency departments are not created equal, you'll want to find out the strengths and weaknesses of your nearest emergency department.

Emergency departments differ in the number of staff they have on hand, the skills of their personnel, and the equipment they have at their disposal.

Emergency physicians are trained to treat all types of emergencies and are involved in all aspects of the EMS system, including training rescue personnel. In 1979, emergency medicine became the twenty-third specialty to be recognized by the American Board of Medical Specialties. In 1991, there were 10,000 board-certified emergency physicians in the United States — not nearly enough for all the emergency facilities in the nation.

Emergency nurses are part of the team in most emergency facilities. They are also active and important members of the EMS system. Emergency nursing is a special area of training and certification for nurses.

Hospitals often focus on one area of critical care, becoming, for example, trauma centers, burn centers, or cardiac centers. This specialization will have a definite impact on a hospital's emergency department. Ask your physician about specialized facilities in your area.

Getting There

If the EMS system has been called, they will transport the victim to an emergency department. Depending upon the circumstances, you may accompany him or her in the ambulance or you may drive to the hospital separately.

If the EMS system has not been dispatched, or if an ambulance is not available, you may have to drive the victim to the nearest emergency department (or other emergency facility) yourself. This is especially true in remote parts of the country. Since you don't want to take unnecessary risks, it's best to seek medical advice before making the decision to drive the victim anywhere yourself. If at all possible, bring along a helper to tend to the victim while you drive. He or she may be needed should the victim's condition worsen.

What to Expect

There is no such thing as a typical emergency department. However, there are typical procedures emergency departments use.

No hospital emergency department can refuse a patient for initial stabilizing treatment of a medical emergency. In every emergency department, patients receive care according to how severe their injuries are, not according to the time they arrive. Don't be surprised if you have to wait while more urgent cases are treated.

Let's assume you are accompanying a family member—your father—who has been injured. As soon as the patient arrives, he is met by a medical professional who makes a brief evaluation of the emergency before your father is registered. The patient will be asked questions to create a medical record. He will also be asked to sign a consent form allowing the emergency department staff to treat him. If the patient is unable to complete this paperwork, a relative will need to do so.

The patient will be taken to an examination room when one becomes available. You may or may not be able to accompany him. If you are allowed to go along, try to make sure the patient's questions are answered and that he understands any procedures or tests that are administered. If either of you is unclear about what is being done, ask questions. If the patient is unconscious, you may find yourself acting as his advocate.

In the course of the care and evaluation, you will meet various support staff. Depending upon the circumstances, these personnel — lab technicians, respiratory therapists, and so forth — will assist in gathering information and giving specialized care.

If the patient requires no more immediate medical treatment, he will be discharged for follow-up care with a private physician, meaning he can go home. The physician will give written discharge instructions and perhaps a prescription for a medication to take. An emergency staff member will review the instructions with you and will include medical advice about the patient's activities. If the patient doesn't have a private physician, he will be referred to one for follow-up care.

Again, these are usual and customary procedures.

You and Your Health Insurance Program

Several million Americans subscribe to health care organizations for their health insurance. These programs often offer emergency care at specific emergency facilities. If you belong to such a health insurance program, become familiar with and be sure to clearly understand its procedures for obtaining emergency medical care. But always remember that any person with a life- or limb-threatening emergency may be initially treated and stabilized in any emergency facility.

First Aid

This section is divided into entries that give you the information you need to provide first aid in most of the situations that come up around the home and workplace. Arranged alphabetically, they range from the minor — **Bites and Stings** — to the serious — **Spinal Injury.** The entries also tell you when to seek medical help. In a few cases we have developed entries for conditions that may be caused by a number of things — **Unconsciousness** and **Bleeding,** for example.

At the beginning of each entry, you'll find important information about the topic. It will help you decide if you're at the right entry, and where to look if you're not. Then you'll find a section called Signs and Symptoms. This list of conditions helps you identify an illness or injury. You should know that a person may show one or all of the signs and symptoms. Next is First Aid, which gives you step-by-step instructions and some important things not to do. More on the Subject is key information related to the emergency—signs of infection or cautions, for example.

At the end of Part 2 you'll find Emergency Action Guides. These quick references for lifesaving techniques cover choking, CPR, and how to control bleeding. They are printed again in the back of the book as tear-outs that you can post on your refrigerator, near your desk at work, or wherever you feel you may need them.

Please read through Part 2 today — before you're faced with an emergency. You'll be familiar with it when you need to use it FAST.

And remember, when an emergency does happen, use your common sense and this book, don't do more than you're comfortable with, and know how to get emergency help.

Find It Fast

Use the expanded list below to help you find the right entry. It lists common terms for first aid emergencies and directs you to the correct entry. In this list, the entry names are in bold type.

Abdominal pain. *See Bleeding.*
Abdominal thrusts. *See Choking.*

Airway, obstructed. *See Choking.*

Alcohol abuse. *See Drug Abuse.*

Allergic Reaction

Amputation

Anaphylaxis. *See Allergic Reaction.*

Angina. *See Heart Attack.*

Ankle injury. *See Bone, Joint, and Muscle Injuries.*

Arm injury. *See Bone, Joint, and Muscle Injuries.*

Arrest, cardiopulmonary. *See Cardiopulmonary Arrest.*

Arrest, respiratory. *See Cardiopulmonary Arrest.*

Baby, birth of. *See Childbirth.*

Back injury. *See Spinal Injury.*

Birth. *See Childbirth.*

Bites and Stings

Bleeding

Bleeding, from mouth. *See Facial Injury.*

Bone, Joint, and Muscle Injuries

Botulism. *See Poison.*

Breathing Problems

Broken bone. *See Bone, Joint, and Muscle Injuries.*

Bruises. *See Bleeding.*

Burn, eye. *See Eye Injury.*

Burn, chemical. *See Chemical Exposure.*

Burns

Cardiopulmonary Arrest. *See also Heart Attack.*

Chemical Exposure

Chemicals, inhaled. *See Poison.*

Chemicals, swallowed. *See Poison.*

Chest pain. *See Heart Attack.*

Chest thrusts. *See Choking.*

Childbirth

Choking

Cold Exposure

Collarbone injury. *See Bone, Joint, and Muscle Injuries.*

Concussion. *See Head Injury.*

Convulsions. *See Seizures.*

CPR. *See Cardiopulmonary Arrest.*

Cramp, muscle. *See Bone, Joint, and Muscle Injuries.*

Cramps. *See Heat Illnesses.*

Croup. *See Breathing Problems.*

Cuts and tears (lacerations). *See Wounds.*

Delivery, of child. *See Childbirth.*

Dental injuries. *See Facial Injury.*

Diabetic reaction. *See Unconsciousness.*

Difficulty breathing. *See Breathing Problems.*

Dislocations. *See Bone, Joint, and Muscle Injuries.*

Dizziness. *See Unconsciousness.*

Drowning

Drug Abuse

Ear Injury

Elbow injury. *See Bone, Joint, and Muscle Injuries.*

Electrical Injury

Electrocution. *See Electrical Injury.*

Epilepsy. *See Seizures.*

Exhaustion, heat. *See Heat Illnesses.*

Exposure, cold. *See Cold Exposure.*

Eye Injury

Facial Injury

Fainting. *See Unconsciousness.*

Fever. *See Seizures.*

Finger injury. *See Bone, Joint, and Muscle Injuries.*

Food poisoning. *See Poison.*

Foot injury. *See Bone, Joint, and Muscle Injuries.*

Fracture. *See Bone, Joint, and Muscle Injuries.*

Fractured skull. *See Head Injury.*

Frostbite. *See Cold Exposure.*

Gagging. *See Choking.*

Gasping. *See Breathing Problems.*

Genital Injury

Hand injury. *See Bone, Joint, and Muscle Injuries.*

Head Injury

Heart Attack. *See also Cardiopulmonary Arrest.*

Heartbeat, irregular. *See Heart Attack.*

Heartbeat, lack of. *See Cardiopulmonary Arrest.*

Heat cramps. *See Heat Illnesses.*

Heat Illnesses

Heatstroke. *See Heat Illnesses.*

Heimlich maneuver. *See Choking.*

Hemorrhage. *See Bleeding.*

Hip injury. *See Bone, Joint, and Muscle Injuries.*

Hives. *See Allergic Reaction.*

Hypothermia. *See Cold Exposure.*

Inhalation poisoning. *See Poison.*

Insect, bites/stings. *See Bites and Stings.*

Insect, in ear. *See Ear Injury.*

Insulin reaction. *See Unconsciousness.*

Internal bleeding. *See Bleeding.*

Jaw injury. *See Facial Injury.*

Joint injuries. *See Bone, Joint, and Muscle Injuries.*

Knee injuries. *See Bone, Joint, and Muscle Injuries.*

Lacerations. *See Wounds.*

Leg injury. *See Bone, Joint, and Muscle Injuries.*

Ligaments, torn. *See Bone, Joint, and Muscle Injuries.*

Mouth injury. *See Facial Injury.*

Mouth-to-mouth resuscitation. *See Cardiopulmonary Arrest.*

Muscle cramps. *See Bone, Joint, and Muscle Injuries.*

Muscle injuries. *See Bone, Joint, and Muscle Injuries.*

Muscles, stiff. *See Bone, Joint, and Muscle Injuries.*

Myocardial infarction. *See Heart Attack.*

Neck injury. *See Spinal Injury.*

Nose Injury

Nosebleeds. *See Nose Injury.*

Overdose, drug or alcohol. *See Drug Abuse.*

Palpitations, heart. *See Heart Attack.*

Pelvis injury. *See Bone, Joint, and Muscle Injuries.*

Poison

Pulse, lack of. *See Cardiopulmonary Arrest.*

Rabies. *See Bites and Stings.*

Rescue, drowning victim. *See Drowning.*

Rescue, ice. *See Drowning.*

Rescue breathing. *See Cardiopulmonary Arrest.*

Respiratory arrest. *See Cardiopulmonary Arrest.*

Rib injury. *See Bone, Joint, and Muscle Injuries.*

Scrapes. *See Wounds.*

Seizures

Shock

Shock, electrical. *See Electrical Injury.*

Shoulder injury. *See Bone, Joint, and Muscle Injuries.*

Skull, injuries to. *See Head Injury.*

Snake bites, nonvenomous. *See Wounds.*

Snake bites, venomous. *See Bites and Stings.*

Spinal Injury

Splinters. *See Wounds.*

Sprains. *See Bone, Joint, and Muscle Injuries.*

Stings. *See Bites and Stings.*

Stroke

Substance abuse. *See Drug Abuse.*

Teeth, loose, broken, or missing. *See Facial Injury.*

Tendon, severed. *See Bone, Joint, and Muscle Injuries.*

Tendonitis. *See Bone, Joint, and Muscle Injuries.*

Toe injury. *See Bone, Joint, and Muscle Injuries.*

Unconsciousness

Urine, blood in. *See Bleeding.*

Vomit, blood in. *See Bleeding.*

Vomiting. *See Head Injury.*

Withdrawal, drug or alcohol. *See Drug Abuse.*

Wounds

Wrist injury. *See Bone, Joint, and Muscle Injuries.*

Zipper injury. *See Wounds.*

Abdominal Pain   *See Bleeding*

Alcohol Abuse   *See Drug Abuse*

Allergic Reaction

Allergies are a type of hypersensitivity. An allergic reaction is the body's defensive response to a substance that is usually harmless. You can be exposed to these substances, called *allergens,* through skin contact, inhalation (breathing), ingestion (swallowing), or injection.

An endless array of substances that don't bother most of us — including the venom from bee stings as well as various foods, pollens, and medications — can trigger allergic reactions in some people. Although you may have no reaction or only a mild reaction the first time you're exposed to an allergen, repeated exposures may lead to more serious reactions. Once you're sensitized, even a very limited exposure to an allergen can trigger a severe reaction. If you know you have serious allergies, you should wear a medical ID tag.

Allergic reactions range from mild to serious and can be localized or general, immediate or delayed (Figure 1). An *anaphylactic reaction* is an allergic reaction that occurs over time; it can last from a few hours to several weeks after you're exposed to an allergen. *Anaphylaxis* is a sudden and severe allergic reaction that occurs within minutes of exposure, progresses rapidly, and can lead to *anaphylactic shock* and death within 15 minutes if medical intervention is not obtained.

Signs and Symptoms

- Itching
- Hives
- Flushed face
- Fear
- Dizziness; weakness
- Swelling of the eyes, face, or tongue
- Nausea; vomiting
- Abdominal cramps or pain
- Difficulty breathing; wheezing; chest tightness
- Difficulty swallowing
- Unconsciousness

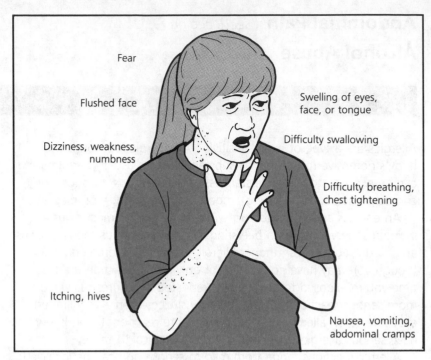

Figure 1
Signs and symptoms of allergic reaction

FIRST AID

Mild to Moderate Allergic Reaction
(Anaphylactic Reaction)

DO NOT assume that any allergy shots the victim has already received will give him or her complete protection.

1. Calm and reassure the victim. Anxiety aggravates all reactions.

2. Try to identify the allergen and have the victim avoid further contact with it. If the allergic reaction is from a honey bee sting, scrape the stinger off the skin with something firm (for example, a fingernail or credit card). *Do not* use tweezers; squeezing the stinger will release more venom.

3. If the victim develops an itchy rash, apply calamine lotion and cool compresses.

4. Monitor the victim for increasing distress.

5. Get medical help. For a mild reaction, a physician may recommend over-the-counter medications.

Severe Allergic Reaction
(Anaphylaxis)

- If the victim's allergic reaction is severe or rapidly worsening, call EMS.
- If the victim has a history of allergic reactions (check for a medical ID tag), call EMS.
- If the victim has emergency allergy medication, help him or her take it.

DO NOT assume that any allergy shots the victim has already received will give him or her complete protection.

DO NOT place a pillow under the victim's head if he or she is having trouble breathing. This can close the airway.

DO NOT give the victim anything by mouth if the victim is having breathing difficulty.

1. Check the victim's ABCs. Open the airway; check breathing and circulation. If necessary, begin rescue breathing, CPR, or bleeding control. (See the Emergency Action Guides on pages 199–210.)

2. Calm and reassure the victim. Anxiety aggravates all reactions.

3. If the allergic reaction is from a honey bee sting, scrape the stinger off the skin with something firm (for example, a fingernail or credit card). *Do not* use tweezers; squeezing the stinger will release more venom.

4. If the victim has emergency allergy medication on hand, help him or her take it. (Some highly sensitive people carry a kit. With the individual's permission, you can help him or her follow the kit instructions.)

5. Take steps to prevent shock. Lay the victim flat, raise his or her feet 8 to 12 inches, and cover the victim with a coat or blanket. *Do not* place the victim in this position if you suspect any head, neck, back, or leg injury or if the position makes the victim uncomfortable. (See **Shock** on page 172.)

6. If the victim loses consciousness, give first aid for unconsciousness until you have medical help. (See **Unconsciousness** on page 182.)

See also **Bites and Stings.**

Amputation is the partial or complete severing of a body part, such as an ear, finger, arm, foot, or leg. Sometimes these parts can be reattached, especially when you take proper care of the severed part and stump.

Signs and Symptoms

- A body part that has been completely cut off
- Crushed body tissue (badly mangled but still partially attached by muscle, bone, tendon, or skin)
- Bleeding (may be minimal or severe, depending on the location and nature of the injury)
- Pain (degree of pain not always related to severity of injury or amount of bleeding)

FIRST AID

Amputation

- Call EMS.
- First, administer first aid for any life-threatening conditions (for example, severe bleeding). Then administer first aid for any other injuries.
- Find and save the severed body parts (see box). It may be possible to reattach them or use them during repair. Be careful to do no further harm to the parts or to the stump.

DO NOT forget that saving the victim's life is more important than saving a body part.

DO NOT overlook other, less obvious, injuries.

DO NOT attempt to push any part back into place.

DO NOT decide that a body part is too small to save.

DO NOT raise false hopes of reattachment.

1. Check the victim's ABCs. Open the airway; check breathing and circulation. If necessary, begin rescue breathing, CPR, or bleeding control. (See the Emergency Action Guides on pages 199–210.)

2. Calm and reassure the victim. Amputation is painful and extremely frightening.

How to Save an Amputated Part

After you give first aid to the victim, try to find and save any severed body parts. It is important to bring an amputated part to the hospital; it may be used to repair the wound.

- Gently rinse any obvious debris off the part.
- See if any ice is readily available.

  If ice is available, wrap the part in a moistened dressing (a clean towel, washcloth, or gauze will do). Place the wrapped part in a plastic bag or sealed container, then place it on a bed of ice and water. Cooling the part will keep it viable for about 18 hours. *Do not* use dry ice, and *do not* place the part directly on the ice.

  If ice is not available, place the part directly in a plastic bag or sealed container without wrapping it in a dressing. The part will remain viable for about 4 to 6 hours.

- Label the container holding the part with the victim's name and the time of the accident.
- Keep the part with the victim. Do not take it to the hospital separately.

3. Control bleeding by applying direct pressure to the wound; by elevating the injured area; and, if necessary, by using pressure point bleeding control. (See **Bleeding** on page 62.)

4. Save and keep with the patient any severed body parts. (See box.)

5. Take steps to prevent shock. Lay the victim flat, raise his or her feet 8 to 12 inches, and cover the victim with a coat or blanket. *Do not* place the victim in this position if you suspect any head, neck, back, or leg injury or if the position makes the victim uncomfortable. (See **Shock** on page 172.)

6. Stay with the victim until you have medical help.

Arm Injury   *See Bone, Joint, and Muscle Injuries*

Back Injury   *See Spinal Injury*

Bites and Stings

"Bites and stings" covers a wide range of conditions, from a single mosquito bite to a serious dog bite. All bites and stings need some wound care to prevent infection. Which first aid measures you should take depends on how severe an injury you have and what bit or stung you. You should know that you can have a severe reaction from a fairly small bite or sting.

Most bites and stings do not require emergency medical attention. But even if you don't need immediate medical care, complications such as delayed allergic reaction, infection at the site, or disease can develop later. Both animals and insects can transmit a variety of potentially serious diseases, including rabies, tetanus, malaria, yellow fever, cat-scratch fever, encephalitis, Rocky Mountain spotted fever, and Lyme disease. Whether or not there is cause for concern depends upon many factors, including what bit or stung you, which diseases are present in the area, and the time of year. Consult a physician for advice.

If there is a severe allergic reaction to a bite or sting, see **Allergic Reaction** on page 45.

For nonvenomous snake bites, see **Wounds** on page 186.

Signs and Symptoms

- An obvious bite, sting, or wound
- A stinger visible in the skin
- Localized pain, redness, itching, swelling, blistering, or burning sensation
- Puncture marks

Possible complications include the following:

- *Reaction to venom.* Signs and symptoms include increasing pain at the site, numbness, tingling, slurred speech, weakness, difficulty breathing, nausea, sweating, and restlessness. The reaction depends on how severe the bite was; the type of venom; the amount of venom and where it was injected; what steps can be taken to prevent the venom from spreading through the body;

and the victim's age, size, general health, and sensitivity to the venom. Children and older people (especially those with chronic health problems) have more severe reactions.

- *Severe allergic reaction.* Signs and symptoms include dizziness; weakness; nausea; vomiting; difficulty breathing or swallowing; a flushed, swollen face; a swollen tongue; hives; or itching. A severe allergic reaction can develop within moments and can be life-threatening. Allergic reaction can also be delayed.
- *Toxic reaction.* This can occur when there are multiple bites or stings. Signs and symptoms include headache, fever, muscle cramps (including abdominal pain), drowsiness, and unconsciousness.
- *Shock.* Signs and symptoms include pale, clammy skin; weakness; bluish lips and fingernails; and decreasing alertness. Shock can be life-threatening.

Insect Stings

FIRST AID

Stinging insects include the bumblebee, honey bee, hornet, yellow jacket, wasp, and fire ant. Only the honey bee leaves its stinger in the skin.

- If the victim is having a severe reaction, call EMS.
- If the victim has been stung inside the mouth or throat, call EMS.
- Try to identify the insect. If it can be done quickly and without danger to you, kill it and have it identified.

1. Check the victim's ABCs. Open the airway; check breathing and circulation. If necessary, begin rescue breathing, CPR, or bleeding control. (See the Emergency Action Guides on pages 199–210.)

2. If the victim is having breathing problems, keep his or her airway open. *Do not* let the victim lie down. A conscious victim will naturally get into the position in which it is easiest to breathe.

3. Calm and reassure the victim. Anxiety aggravates all reactions.

4. If the victim was stung by a honey bee, remove the stinger from the skin by scraping it off with something firm (for example, a fingernail or credit card). *Do not* use tweezers; pinching the stinger will release more venom.

5. Wash the sting(s) with soap and water to help prevent infection. Then apply a cold compress to reduce the pain and swelling and to slow the spread of the venom.

6. Remove any rings or constricting items, since the injured area may swell.

7. If the victim develops an allergic reaction, give first aid for allergic reaction. (See page 45.)

8. If the victim received multiple stings, watch for a severe allergic reaction.

9. Stay with the victim for at least an hour after the sting occurred and continue to monitor ABCs.

More on the Subject

Make sure the victim is up to date on tetanus immunizations. If signs of infection develop — including increased pain, redness, swelling, discharge, swollen lymph nodes, fever, or red streaks spreading from the site toward the heart — get medical help immediately.

FIRST AID

Insect Bites

Biting insects include fleas, mosquitoes, bedbugs, lice, chiggers, and gnats. These insects are not poisonous, but their bites sometimes lead to complications.

1. Wash the bite with soap and water to help prevent infection.

2. If there is pain and irritation at the site of the bite, apply a cold compress or an antiseptic or anesthetic ointment.

More on the Subject

Make sure the victim is up to date on tetanus immunizations. Signs and symptoms of illness may develop days after the bite occurred. If signs of infection develop — including increased pain, redness, swelling, discharge, swollen lymph nodes, fever, or red streaks spreading from the site toward the heart — get medical help immediately.

FIRST AID

Tick Bites

Ticks burrow into the skin and suck blood from their host. They can transmit Rocky Mountain spotted fever, Colorado tick fever, Lyme disease, and other illnesses. Some ticks inject a venom that causes tick paralysis, but only as long as the tick remains attached in the skin.

1. Don't forcefully pull off a tick that is attached in the skin; you might pull off the body but leave the head. Instead, suffocate the tick by covering it with petroleum jelly, mineral oil, or some other heavy oil. The tick may release at once. If not, wait half an hour, then pull it off carefully with tweezers, grasping as close as possible to the mouth part of the tick. Make sure all parts of the tick are completely removed.

2. Wash the bite with soap and water to help prevent infection.

3. If you can't remove all parts of the tick, get medical help.

More on the Subject

Make sure the victim is up to date on tetanus immunizations. Signs and symptoms of illness may develop days, weeks, or months after the bite occurred. If signs of infection develop — including increased pain, redness, swelling, discharge, swollen lymph nodes, fever, flu-like symptoms, or red streaks spreading from the site toward the heart — get medical help immediately.

Venomous Spider and Scorpion Bites

Most spider bites are not a cause for concern. However, a bite from a black widow spider, brown recluse spider, tarantula, or scorpion may be venomous (see box on page 54) and requires immediate first aid followed by medical help.

- If the victim is having a severe reaction, call EMS.
- Try to identify the spider or scorpion. If it can be done quickly and without danger to you, kill it and have it identified.
- Call ahead to the emergency department so the correct antivenin can be prepared.

DO NOT apply a tourniquet.
DO NOT raise the site of the bite above the level of the victim's heart.
DO NOT give the victim aspirin, stimulants, or pain medication unless a physician says to.
DO NOT allow the victim to exercise. If necessary, carry him or her to safety.

1. Check the victim's ABCs. Open the airway; check breathing and circulation. If necessary, begin rescue breathing, CPR, or bleeding control. (See the Emergency Action Guides on pages 199–210.)

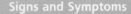

By familiarizing yourself with the descriptions that follow, you will be able to recognize a potentially deadly scorpion or spider.

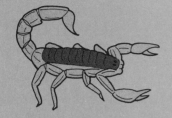

Scorpion

A scorpion looks like a little lobster with 8 legs and a flexible tail with a stinger on the end. All scorpions are venomous, and some scorpions' venom can be fatal.

Signs and Symptoms

There is immediate pain at the sting site. If the site is on an arm or leg, burning and tingling may spread up the limb. Restlessness and difficulty with vision and speech may occur. Seizure-like shaking may develop.

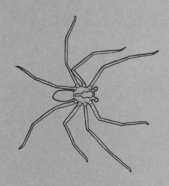

Black Widow

The black widow spider actually can be either black or brown and has a red hourglass shape on its underside. The male black widow is usually too small to inflict a serious bite.

Venom affects the nervous system and can cause muscle spasms and cramps, nausea, vomiting, and difficulty breathing, anywhere from 1 to 24 hours after the bite occurs.

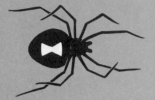

Brown Recluse

The brown recluse spider is tan or yellow-brown and has a dark violin-shaped mark on its back.

Venom causes local tissue damage. A painless ulcer at the site continues to enlarge and is slow to heal. Chills, aches, and nausea may occur in the first few hours.

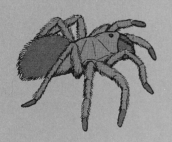

Tarantula

The tarantula is very large and hairy. Tarantulas do not always inject venom into their victims, but even minor bites can cause considerable tissue damage.

Tarantula bites usually do not produce generalized reactions, but they can cause local damage. A bite can produce a painful sore that takes up to several weeks to heal.

2. Calm and reassure the victim. Anxiety aggravates all reactions.

3. If the victim is having breathing problems, keep his or her airway open. A conscious victim will naturally get into the position in which it is easiest to breathe.

4. Wash the bite or sting with soap and water to help prevent infection. Then apply a cold compress to reduce the pain and swelling and to slow the spread of the venom.

5. Remove any rings or constricting items, since the bitten area may swell.

6. Take steps to slow the rate at which the venom spreads in the victim's body. Have the victim stay still. Place the injured site below the level of the victim's heart and immobilize the injured site in a comfortable position.

7. Look for signs of shock, such as decreased alertness and increased paleness. If shock develops, lay the victim flat, raise his or her feet 8 to 12 inches, and cover the victim with a coat or blanket. *Do not* elevate the bitten area, and *do not* place the victim in this position if you suspect any head, neck, back, or leg injury or if the position makes the victim uncomfortable. (See **Shock** on page 172.)

8. Stay with the victim until you have medical help and monitor ABCs.

More on the Subject

Make sure the victim is up to date on tetanus immunizations. Venomous bites can cause severe local tissue damage and often require follow-up care by a physician. If signs of infection develop — including increased pain, redness, swelling, discharge, swollen lymph nodes, fever, or red streaks spreading from the site toward the heart — get medical help immediately.

How to Recognize Venomous Snakes in North America

Most snakes in North America are not venomous. The two types of poisonous snakes you should be aware of, pit vipers and coral snakes, are described in this chart.

Pit Vipers

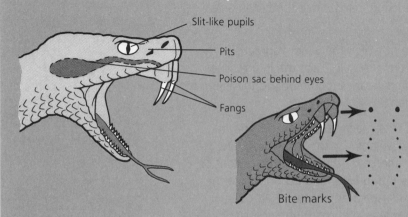

Slit-like pupils

Pits

Poison sac behind eyes

Fangs

Bite marks

Rattlesnakes, copperheads, and cottonmouths are all *pit vipers.* You can recognize a pit viper by its triangular head, fangs, narrow, vertical pupils, and the pits between its nostrils and its eyes. The coral snake has round pupils and is not a pit viper; it does have fangs, but they may or may not be visible. Nonvenomous snakes have round pupils and no fangs, pits, or rattles.

Bite Marks
A pit viper punctures its victim with fangs. There may be one or more puncture marks.

Signs and Symptoms
Venom affects the circulatory system. Signs and symptoms include immediate pain at the site of the bite that becomes more severe, rapid swelling and discoloration at the site of the bite, dizziness, nausea, sweating, headache, thirst, difficulty breathing, and shock.

FIRST AID

Venomous Snake Bites

A bite from a nonvenomous snake should be treated as a wound. (See **Wounds** on page 186.) A bite from a venomous snake requires immediate first aid followed by medical help.

In North America there are 2 types of venomous snakes (see box), plus 2 venomous lizards: the gila monster and the beaded lizard. If there is any doubt about whether or not a bite was caused by a venomous snake or lizard, play it safe and assume it was.

It usually takes several hours for snake venom to kill. The correct antivenin can save your life if it is administered promptly.

Rattlesnake

Rattlers grow up to 8 feet long. These are about 30 species of rattlesnake in the U.S., but any rattler can be recognized by the rattles at the end of its tail.

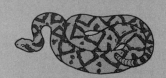

Copperhead

Copperheads grow up to 4 feet long and have diamond-shaped markings down their backs. They vibrate their tails when angry, but have no rattles.

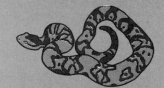

Cottonmouth

The cottonmouth, also known as the water moccasin, grows up to 4 feet long. When alarmed, it opens its mouth, revealing the white lining for which it is named.

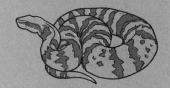

Coral Snake

Coral snakes grow up to 3 feet long and have distinctive red, black, and yellow or white rings and a black nose. Other snakes have similar colors, but only the coral snake has red bands bordered by white or yellow.

Bite Marks

The coral snake chews its victim to inject its venom. It may leave tooth marks with or without fang puncture marks.

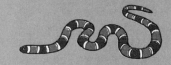

Signs and Symptoms

Venom affects the nervous system. Signs and symptoms include minor pain at site of bite, droopy eyelids, drowsiness, slurred speech, double vision, drooling, sweating, nausea, delirium, and convulsions.

- Call EMS.
- Try to identify the type of snake. If it can be done quickly and without danger to you, kill the snake and have it identified. (Be aware that venomous snakes can bite reflexively even after they die.)
- Call ahead to the emergency department so the correct anti-venin can be prepared.

Rabies

Rabies is a rare but potentially fatal disease transmitted by the saliva of a rabid animal (bat, skunk, raccoon, fox, squirrel, dog, etc.).

There are only two ways to tell whether or not an animal is rabid: by capturing the animal and placing it under observation for 10 days, or by killing it and having its brain examined for signs of the disease. Don't go near an animal that may be rabid. Notify the proper authorities (police or animal control) if you are bitten by a wild animal or by a domestic animal if you can't immediately find out if it has been vaccinated against rabies. Tell them what the animal looks like and where it is so they can capture it.

There is no cure for rabies once you develop symptoms, but if you're vaccinated promptly after being exposed to the disease, you can develop immunity before symptoms develop. Whether or not you need to be treated for rabies depends upon many factors. A physician must make the decision.

DO NOT cut into a snake bite.

DO NOT apply cold compresses to a snake bite.

DO NOT apply a tourniquet.

DO NOT raise the site of the bite above the level of the victim's heart.

DO NOT give the victim aspirin, stimulants, or pain medication unless a physician says to.

DO NOT allow the victim to exercise. If necessary, carry him or her to safety.

1. Check the victim's ABCs. Open the airway; check breathing and circulation. If necessary, begin rescue breathing, CPR, or bleeding control. (See the Emergency Action Guides on pages 199–210.)

2. If the victim is having breathing problems, keep his or her airway open. A conscious victim will naturally get into the position in which it is easiest to breathe.

3. Calm and reassure the victim. Anxiety aggravates all reactions.

4. Wash the bite with soap and water.

5. Remove any rings or constricting items, since the bitten area may swell.

6. Take steps to slow the rate at which the venom spreads in the victim's body. Have the victim lie still. Place the injured site below the level of the victim's heart and immobilize it in a comfortable position.

7. Look for signs of shock, such as decreased alertness or increased paleness. If shock develops, lay the victim flat, raise his or her feet 8 to 12 inches, and cover the victim with a coat or blanket. *Do not* elevate the bitten area, and *do not* place the victim in this position if you suspect any head, neck, back, or leg injury or if the position makes the victim uncomfortable. (See **Shock** on page 172.)

8. Stay with the victim until you get medical help.

More on the Subject

Venomous bites can cause severe local tissue damage and often require follow-up care. If signs of infection develop — including increased pain, redness, swelling, discharge, swollen lymph nodes, fever, or red streaks spreading from the site toward the heart — get medical help immediately. It is important for everyone to be up to date on tetanus immunization. If you are in an area with poisonous snakes, carry a snakebite kit and know how to use it.

Animal and Human Bites

If you have an animal or a human bite, you generally need medical attention because of the likelihood of infection.

- If the victim has been seriously wounded, call EMS.
- If the victim was bitten by an animal, you will need to contact authorities so they can find out whether or not the animal was rabid. (See box.)

1. Calm and reassure the victim. Put on latex gloves or wash your hands.

2. Check for bleeding.

    If the bite is not bleeding severely, wash it well (for at least 5 minutes) with mild soap and running water, then apply a bandage. (See **Wounds** on page 186.)

    If the bite is actively bleeding, control bleeding by applying direct pressure to the bite; by elevating the injured area; and, if necessary, by using pressure point bleeding control. (See **Bleeding** on page 62.) *Do not* attempt to clean a wound that is actively bleeding.

3. Get medical help.

More on the Subject

If signs of infection develop — including increased pain, redness, swelling, discharge, swollen lymph nodes, fever, or red streaks spreading from the site toward the heart — get medical help immediately. Everyone should be up to date on tetanus immunization.

Poisonous Marine Life

There are many types of venomous creatures in the ocean, and they deliver venom in a variety of ways. Antivenins exist for some, but not all, marine venoms.

- If the victim is having a severe reaction, call EMS.
- Try to determine the cause of the bite or sting. If it can be done quickly and without danger to you, kill the creature and have it identified.

■ Call ahead to the emergency department so the correct antivenin (if one exists) can be prepared.

DO NOT raise a venomous bite above the level of the victim's heart.
DO NOT give the victim aspirin, stimulants, or pain medication unless a physician says to.
DO NOT allow the victim to exercise. If necessary, carry him or her to safety.

1. Calm and reassure the victim. Anxiety aggravates all reactions.

2. Check the victim's ABCs. Open the airway; check breathing and circulation. If necessary, begin rescue breathing, CPR, or bleeding control. (See the Emergency Action Guides on pages 199–210.)

3. If the victim is having breathing problems, keep his or her airway open. A conscious victim will naturally get into the position in which it is easiest to breathe.

4. Check for bleeding.
   If there is no severe bleeding, clean the wound and rinse it well with salt water. Marine wounds need to be thoroughly cleaned to remove contaminants such as sand, spines, shell fragments, bristles, pieces of coral, or even teeth. Proper cleaning of the wound may have to be done by a physician.
   If there is severe bleeding, control bleeding by applying direct pressure to the wound and, if necessary, by using pressure point bleeding control. (See **Bleeding** on page 62.)

5. Remove any rings or constricting items, since the injured area may swell.

6. Bandage the injured area. (See **Wounds** on page 186.)

7. Take steps to slow the rate at which the venom spreads in the victim's body. Have the victim stay still. Place the injured site below the level of the victim's heart and immobilize it in a comfortable position.

8. Take steps to prevent shock. Lay the victim flat, raise his or her feet 8 to 12 inches, and cover the victim with a coat or blanket. *Do not* elevate the injured area, and *do not* place the victim in this position if you suspect head, neck, back, or leg injury or if the position causes the victim discomfort.

9. Stay with the victim until you get medical help and continue to monitor ABCs.

First Aid for Specific Marine Life Injuries

Bristleworm. Remove dry stinging bristles with adhesive tape. Then apply rubbing alcohol or a solution of 1 part household ammonia to 4 parts water.

Cone shell. Cone shells inject their venom through a puncture wound. Soak the wound in hot water for at least 30 minutes.

Fire coral. Fire coral injects its venom through stinging cells and produces multiple sharp cuts. Give first aid for wounds.

Jellyfish and the Portuguese man-of-war. Jellyfish deliver their venom through stinging cells on their tentacles. Be careful around fragments of tentacle; they are capable of stinging even after the tentacle is detached from the body of the jellyfish. Try to remove the tentacles by lifting them off with a knife, comb, etc., or, for larger tentacles, forceps or tweezers. Never rub them off, as this will activate more of the stinging cells. Rinse the stings with seawater and soak in vinegar or rubbing alcohol for 30 minutes or until pain is relieved.

Sea snake. Treat as a venomous snake bite. (See page 56.)

Sea urchin. Sea urchins have sharp spines that often get stuck in the skin. Remove any readily visible spines, but get medical help for removal of spines near a joint. Soaking in hot (110° to 113° Fahrenheit) water frequently relieves pain.

Sting ray. The sting ray can both cut and puncture its victim. Rinse the wound with water, preferably seawater, to remove the venom and immediately soak the wound in water as hot as the victim can tolerate for 30 to 90 minutes or until pain is relieved. Apply a dry dressing and get medical help.

Stinging fish (scorpion fish). Soak the sting in water as hot as the victim can tolerate for 30 to 90 minutes or until pain is relieved. Get medical help.

More on the Subject

Deeply buried fragments often must be located by X ray and removed by a physician.

Venomous bites can cause severe local tissue damage. As a preventive measure, your physician may prescribe antibiotics. If signs of infection develop — including increased pain, redness, swelling, discharge, swollen lymph nodes, fever, or red streaks spreading from the site toward the heart — get medical help immediately. Make sure the victim is up to date on tetanus immunizations.

Bleeding

Damage to a blood vessel causes bleeding, which can range from minor to life-threatening. *Bruises* form when blood leaks into tissue beneath the skin. *External bleeding* happens when there's any type of break in the skin. *Internal bleeding* can be caused by illness, injury, or certain medications and it can be difficult to detect.

Internal bleeding often occurs when there has been a broken bone or a blunt or penetrating blow to the body (trauma), particularly to the abdomen.

If any tissue or body part has been torn off, see **Amputation** on page 48.

If the victim has a head injury, see **Head Injury** on page 147.

If the victim has a wound that is not bleeding severely or a wound with an object embedded in it, see **Wounds** on page 186.

If applicable, see **Ear Injury** on page 129, **Eye Injury** on page 136, **Facial Injury** on page 142, **Genital Injury** on page 146, or **Nose Injury** on page 160.

Signs and Symptoms

- Blood coming from an open wound
- Blood in vomit (looks bright red or brown like coffee grounds), in the stool (can appear black or bright red), or in the urine
- Blood coming from the vagina
- Pain and/or swelling of the abdomen
- Bruises
- Weakness; confusion
- Shock. (Signs and symptoms include pale, clammy skin; weakness; bluish lips and fingernails; and decreasing alertness.)

Bruises

Bruises are dark, discolored areas. Sometimes a lump called a *hematoma* forms.

- If you suspect internal bleéding, call EMS.
- If you suspect a broken bone or if there is any loss of function or sensation, get medical help.
- If bruises appear for no apparent reason, get medical help. This can be a sign of serious illness.

1. Apply a cold compress as soon as possible to reduce swelling. *Do not* put ice directly on the skin.

2. If the bruise is on an arm or leg, raise it above the level of the heart to reduce blood flow to the injured area. (If you suspect a spinal injury, do not raise the victim's legs.)

External Bleeding

FIRST AID

Within the body's circulatory system, *arteries* carry oxygen-rich blood from the heart, and *veins* carry used blood back to the heart. *Arterial bleeding* is life-threatening and needs to be controlled immediately; with each beat of the heart more bright red, oxygen-rich blood spurts from the wound. *Venous bleeding* creates a steady flow; it does not spurt like arterial bleeding but can be severe.

The amount of blood is not a good way to judge the severity of an injury. Serious injuries don't always bleed heavily, and some minor injuries (for example, scalp wounds) bleed profusely. Also, the blood of people who take blood-thinning medication or have a bleeding disorder such as hemophilia may not clot easily.

When giving first aid for open wounds, it's important to take precautions to protect against the transmission of disease. It's best to wear sterile gloves. If you have no gloves, put several layers of dressings or a layer of plastic wrap between you and the wound. Always wash your hands before and after you give first aid. (For more information on the transmission of infectious diseases, see Health Precautions and Guidelines for the Rescuer on page 25.)

- If there is severe external bleeding, call EMS.
- Try to identify all sources of bleeding, external and internal.

DO NOT probe a wound or pull out any embedded object from a wound. This will almost certainly cause more bleeding and harm.
DO NOT try to clean a large wound. This can cause heavier bleeding.

DO NOT use a tourniquet.

DO NOT remove a dressing if it becomes soaked with blood. Instead, add a new one on top.

DO NOT peek at a wound to see if the bleeding is stopping. The less a wound is disturbed, the more likely it is that you'll be able to control the bleeding.

DO NOT try to clean a wound after you get bleeding under control. Get medical help.

1. Calm and reassure the victim. The sight of blood can be very frightening.

2. Locate the source of the bleeding.

3. Wash your hands.

4. Put on sterile gloves if you have them. Remove any obvious loose debris from the wound.

5. Using a sterile dressing or clean cloth, apply direct pressure to the wound to stop the bleeding. (See box on page 66.) Direct pressure is almost always appropriate for brisk bleeding; however, *do not* use direct pressure on an eye injury, on a wound that contains an embedded object, or on a head injury if there is a possibility of skull fracture.

6. Raise the bleeding part above the level of the victim's heart *if* you don't suspect a broken bone and if elevating the injury doesn't cause the victim more pain.

7. If the bleeding doesn't stop or if you need to free your hands, apply a pressure bandage. (See box on page 67.)

8. If the bleeding doesn't stop after 15 minutes of direct pressure or if the wound is too extensive to cover effectively, use pressure point bleeding control. (See box on page 68.)

9. If the bleeding stops with direct pressure but then starts up again, reapply direct pressure.

10. If the bleeding is severe, get medical help and take steps to prevent shock. Lay the victim flat, raise his or her feet 8 to 12 inches, and cover the victim with a coat or blanket. *Do not* place the victim in the shock position if you suspect any head, neck, back, or leg injury or if the position makes the victim uncomfortable. (See **Shock** on page 172.)

11. Get medical help if you can't stop the bleeding by yourself. Wounds that need medical attention include deep or jagged wounds; wounds that occur with a broken bone, a loss of function, a loss of sensation, or over joints; gaping wounds; and animal or human bites. (See **Wounds** on page 186.)

More on the Subject

If signs of infection develop — including increased pain, redness, swelling, discharge, swollen lymph nodes, fever, or red streaks spreading from the site toward the heart — get medical help immediately. Make sure the victim is up to date on tetanus immunization.

Internal Bleeding

Internal bleeding can be life-threatening and may need to be treated in a hospital. Sometimes the signs and symptoms of internal bleeding can take days or weeks to appear. Unless the victim is properly examined after major trauma, internal bleeding may go unnoticed until it is too late.

- If you suspect internal bleeding, call EMS.

1. Check the victim's ABCs. Open the airway; check breathing and circulation. If necessary, begin rescue breathing, CPR, or bleeding control. (See the Emergency Action Guides on pages 199–210.)

2. Keep the victim still while you wait for medical help.

3. Do not give the victim anything to eat or drink.

4. Take steps to prevent shock. Lay the victim flat, elevate his or her feet 8 to 12 inches, and cover the victim with a coat or blanket. *Do not* place the victim in the shock position if you suspect any head, neck, back, or leg injury or if the position makes the victim uncomfortable. (See **Shock** on page 172.)

5. If the victim vomits and you do not suspect a spinal injury, place him or her on one side to avoid blocking the airway. (See Vomiting on page 151.) Save the vomit so it can be checked by a physician.

How to Apply Direct Pressure to Stop Bleeding

A minor wound will stop bleeding by itself by forming a clot. With a serious injury, blood may flow from the wound so quickly that it does not have a chance to clot. In this case, your goal is to press hard on the bleeding vessels in order to compress them and allow clots to form. Call EMS whenever bleeding isn't quickly controlled.

To apply direct pressure, do the following (Figure 4):

1. Wear sterile gloves or put several layers of dressings or a layer of plastic wrap over the wound.
2. Place a thick pad of sterile gauze or clean cloth over the wound. If the wound is gaping, press its edges together. If you have no dressing to place over the wound, use a clean cloth or, as a last resort, your hand.
3. Press firmly on the dressing with one hand and elevate the wound higher than the victim's heart.

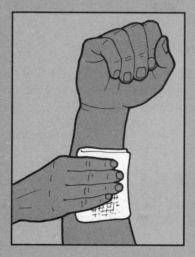

Figure 4
Applying direct pressure to control bleeding

4. If blood soaks through the dressing, *do not* remove it. Apply another dressing on top and keep pressing.
5. If bleeding continues, press harder, using both hands.
6. Continue to apply direct pressure without letting up. If the victim has no history of bleeding problems (for example, hemophilia), direct pressure should stop the bleeding within 15 minutes.
7. If the wound is still bleeding after 15 minutes of continuous direct pressure, continue direct pressure, get medical help, and start pressure point bleeding control. (See box on page 68.)

How to Apply a Pressure Bandage

If the bleeding stops, or if you need to free your hands to attend to other injuries or move the victim, a pressure bandage will hold dressings in place and maintain pressure on the wound.

To apply a pressure bandage, do the following (Figure 5):

1. Hold dressings firmly in place over the wound.
2. Wrap a roller bandage or long strip of cloth firmly around the wound, securing the dressings in place. If the wound is on a limb, use overlapping turns. *Do not* wrap the bandage over and over the same spot.
3. Split the end of the bandage into 2 strips, then tie the ends tight. Tie the knot directly over the wound.

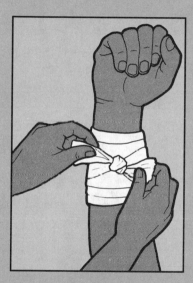

Figure 5
Applying a pressure bandage

4. Check to be sure the pressure bandage is not too tight. It should be tight enough to maintain pressure on the wound, but not so tight that it cuts off circulation further down the arm or leg. If you can't detect a pulse beyond the wound, or if the skin beyond the wound is turning bluish, the pressure bandage is too tight.

(*Note*: Other bandaging techniques are discussed under **Wounds** on page 186.)

How to Use Pressure Point Bleeding Control

If direct pressure and elevation don't control bleeding from an injured arm or leg, call EMS if you have not done so already. The next step is to reduce the flow of blood to the wound. You can do this by compressing the major artery that supplies the injured area with blood. But this technique stops normal circulation within the injured arm or leg, so use it *only when absolutely necessary*.

There's a point on each arm and leg where the artery can be pressed against a bone to interrupt circulation (Figure 6).

- *For an arm wound*, the pressure point is on the *brachial artery* between the large muscles (biceps and triceps) on the inside of the upper arm. Feel for a pulse below the round muscle of the biceps. Then, using 4 fingers, press the artery against the bone until you can no longer feel a pulse.
- *For a leg wound*, the pressure point is on the *femoral artery* in the groin at the top of the leg where the leg bends. Place the victim on his or her back and feel for a pulse in the groin. (If spinal injury is suspected, apply pressure point bleeding control without moving the victim.) Then, using the heel of your hand and keeping your arm straight, press the artery against the pelvic bone. If you need to apply more pressure, use both hands.

Continue using direct pressure and elevation along with pressure point bleeding control. If it is done properly, this technique will almost immediately stop or significantly slow severe bleeding.

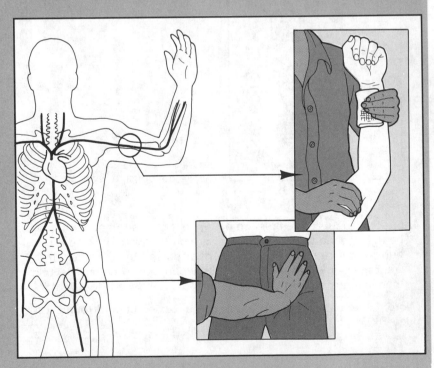

Figure 6
Pressure point bleeding control

When they're all in alignment and working smoothly together, bones, joints, and muscles — known collectively as the *musculoskeletal system* — give the body a framework and allow movement.

The musculoskeletal system has many intricate connections that allow the body to do many different things. *Muscles* expand and contract, enabling you to move. They are attached to bones by their tapered ends, called *tendons*. *Bones* help support the body. They also protect some internal organs. Bones are connected to each other at flexible *joints* by means of *ligaments*. Bone ends are covered with *cartilage* where they meet, and each joint is kept lubricated by thick *synovial fluid* produced by a membrane called the *synovium*, which lines the *joint capsule* around each joint (Figure 7). Illness or injury can affect any of these structures.

Injuries to the bones, joints, or muscles range from minor to severe. Bones, for example, are rigid and can be fractured when they break or split. Muscles and ligaments are made up of many separate fibers, and they can stretch, tear, or snap if overstressed. Medical advice is often needed to diagnose the problem correctly. When in doubt, get medical help.

People tend to ignore or underestimate minor muscle and joint injuries. You should know that a delay in the repair of certain kinds of injuries can lead to permanent loss of function. Also, if minor injuries aren't allowed to fully heal, it's easy to reinjure them, and that could lead to serious lifetime limitations.

If a body part has been cut off or crushed, see **Amputation** on page 48.

If the victim has a broken tooth, broken facial bones, or a broken jaw, see **Facial Injury** on page 142.

If the victim has muscle cramps because of heat illness, see **Heat Illnesses** on page 155.

If you suspect a broken nose, see **Nose Injury** on page 160.

If you suspect a broken neck or back, see **Spinal Injury** on page 175.

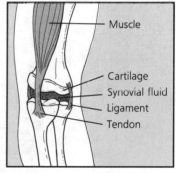

Figure 7
Parts of a joint

Signs and Symptoms

- Pain
- Bruising; discoloration. (Gravity sometimes makes bruises show up some distance from the original injury.)
- Swelling
- Misshapen appearance; obvious deformity. (A limb may appear bent or shortened.)
- Exposed bone
- Pale, bluish skin; loss of pulse in an injured limb. (A serious bone or joint injury keeps blood from flowing properly to points farther down the arm or leg.)
- Numbness farther down the arm or leg

Bone, joint, and muscle injuries include the following:

- *Stiff muscles* are caused by overexertion. They ache and are sore, but there is no loss of function.
- *Tendonitis* is the inflammation of a muscle tendon, usually due to repeated use. It causes mild to severe pain.
- *Muscle cramp* (or spasm) is the sudden, painful tightening of a muscle.
- *Muscle strain*, or pulled muscle, is the sudden, painful tearing of muscle fiber during exertion. Signs and symptoms include pain, swelling, bruising, and loss of efficient movement.
- *Severed tendon* can result from overexertion or a serious cut. There is pain and loss of function.
- *Sprain* occurs when a joint loosens. This is caused by torn fibers in a ligament. Sprains are painful and can cause swelling and bruising, but the joint may still function and usually does not appear misshapen unless all the fibers of a ligament are torn.
- *Joint effusion* occurs when the synovium, due to illness or injury, fills up with blood, synovial fluid (the fluid produced in the synovium to lubricate the joint), or infected fluid. The joint can appear swollen if enough fluid is present.
- *Joint dislocation* can happen when bones come out of alignment. Signs and symptoms include pain, misshapen appearance, swelling, and loss of function.
- *Broken bones* (split or snap). Fractures can be closed (the skin is not broken) or open (one or both bone ends pierce the skin). Signs and symptoms can include pain, swelling, and misshapen appearance. However, a broken bone may not be misshapen or

even very painful, and it is a myth that you cannot use a broken bone. If you have any suspicion that a bone is broken, assume that it is.

Muscle Cramps

Muscle cramps can occur any time — during exertion or at rest. Sometimes they're caused by certain medications or dehydration.

1. Have the victim stretch out the affected muscle to counteract the cramp.

2. Massage the cramped muscle firmly but gently.

3. Apply heat. (Use a heating pad or a hot water bottle wrapped in cloth.) Moist heat is more effective than dry heat. *Do not* apply direct heat to the skin.

4. Get medical help if cramps persist.

Muscle Strains
(Pulled Muscles)

1. Apply cold compresses at once. Reapply them for 20 minutes every 3 to 4 hours for the first 24 hours. (*Do not* apply ice directly to the skin.)

2. If the strained muscle is in an arm or leg, elevate the limb to reduce swelling and bleeding within the muscle. Rest the pulled muscle for 24 hours.

3. Get medical help if the victim is in great pain or if a body part is not working properly.

More on the Subject

If the muscle feels better after 24 hours, apply heat as often as possible for the next 3 to 4 days. *Do not* apply direct heat to the skin. If the problem has not improved in 24 hours, get medical help.

A strained muscle should not be used as long as it is painful. When it is no longer painful, the victim should return to full activity gradually. If the muscle starts to hurt again, reapply heat and slowly start activity.

FIRST AID

Sprains

- If the victim is severely injured or you suspect a broken bone, call EMS. Get medical help if the injured area is misshapen, if the victim is in great pain, if a body part is not working properly, or if there are signs that circulation beyond the injured area has been impaired.

DO NOT give the victim anything by mouth if you suspect severe injury.

DO NOT ignore persistent joint pain. A body part that hurts should not be used.

1. Remove any clothing or jewelry from around the joint.

2. Apply cold compresses at once. Reapply them as often as possible (at least for 20 minutes every 3 to 4 hours) for the first 24 hours. (*Do not* apply ice directly to the skin.)

3. Elevate the affected joint with pillows or clothing. Do not move the injured area for at least 24 hours.

4. The victim's physician may recommend an over-the-counter anti-inflammatory medication (aspirin, ibuprofen) appropriate for the victim's general health.

FIRST AID

Dislocations and Broken Bones

If a joint is overstressed, the bones that meet at that joint may get disconnected, or *dislocated*. When this happens, there's usually a torn joint capsule and torn ligaments, and often, nerve injury.

If more pressure is put on a bone than it can stand, it will fracture (split or break). Open fractures (in which bone pierces the skin) can easily become infected.

If an infant or toddler does not start to use an injured arm or leg within hours of an accident, or if he or she continues to cry when the injured area is touched, assume the child has a broken bone, and get medical help.

It's hard to tell a dislocated bone from a broken bone. Both are an emergency. The general first aid steps are the same for both.

- If you suspect that the victim has a dislocation or broken bone, and there is severe bleeding, call EMS.
- If you cannot completely immobilize the injury at the scene by yourself, call EMS.

DO NOT move the victim unless the injured area is totally immobilized.

DO NOT move a victim with an injured hip, pelvis, or upper leg unless it is absolutely necessary. If you must move the victim immediately, use the clothes drag technique (see page 178).

DO NOT attempt to straighten a misshapen bone or joint or to change its position.

DO NOT test a misshapen bone or joint for loss of function.

DO NOT give the victim anything by mouth.

1. Check the victim's ABCs. Open the airway; check breathing and circulation. If necessary, begin rescue breathing, CPR, or bleeding control. (See the Emergency Action Guides on pages 199–210.)

2. Keep the victim still.

3. If the skin is pierced by a broken bone, or if you suspect there may be a broken bone beneath an open wound, take steps to prevent infection. *Do not* breathe on the wound, and *do not* wash or probe it. Cover it with sterile dressings before immobilizing the injury. (See **Wounds** on page 186.)

4. Splint or sling the injury in the position in which you found it. (See boxes on pages 76 and 77.) It is important to immobilize the area both above and below the injured joint and to check the circulation of the affected area after immobilizing. Guidelines for specific parts of the body are given below.

5. Take steps to prevent shock. Lay the victim flat, elevate his or her feet 8 to 12 inches, and cover the victim with a coat or blanket. *Do not* place the victim in the shock position if you suspect any head, neck, back, or leg injury or if the position causes the victim discomfort.

6. Get medical help.

Ankle. To immobilize an injured ankle, put a pillow or folded blanket underneath the foot and ankle (Figure 8). First wrap one end of the pillow around the ankle and tie it in 2 places; then wrap the other end of the pillow around the toes and tie it in 1 place. Leave the toes exposed. Elevate the ankle.

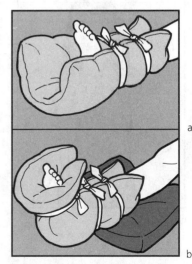

a

b

Figure 8 a, b
Immobilizing an ankle

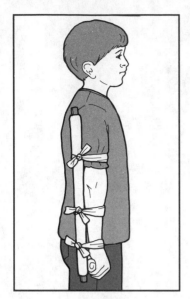

Figure 9
Splinting an elbow that is
already straight

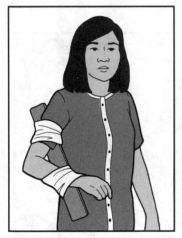

Figure 10
Splinting an elbow that is
already bent

Arm. To immobilize the *upper arm*, apply a sling. Then use another tie to bind the sling across the chest. (See box on page 77.) To immobilize the *forearm* or *wrist*, see Wrist (later in this section).

Collarbone. To immobilize an injured collarbone, apply a sling (see box on page 77) to keep the victim's arm and shoulder blade elevated. Then use another tie to bend the sling across the chest.

Elbow. To immobilize an injured elbow that is already straight, apply a splint (see box on page 76) along the arm and tie it in several places (Figure 9). Do not bend the elbow as you apply the splint.

To immobilize an injured elbow that is already bent, apply a splint diagonally across the underside of the arm (Figure 10). The splint should extend several inches beyond both the upper arm and the wrist.

Finger. Apply cold compresses and elevate the injured hand.

Foot. See Ankle.

Forearm. See Wrist.

Hand. See Wrist.

Hip. Don't move a victim with an injured hip unless absolutely necessary. Wait for medical help to arrive. If you *must* move a victim with an injured hip, you'll need two boards that you have padded with blankets or towels to splint the injured side (Figure 11). Place a long board on the outside of the leg, extending from the armpit to below the heel. Place a second board on the inside of the leg, extending from the groin to below the heel. Secure the splints at the chest, waist, groin, thigh, knee, and ankle.

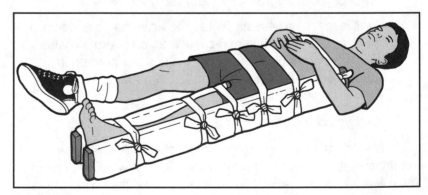

Figure 11
Immobilizing a hip

Knee. To immobilize an injured knee that is already straight, apply a splint as for an injured leg (next). If the injured knee is already bent, don't try to straighten it. Instead, immobilize the injured knee by having the victim bend his or her other knee to the same angle (Figure 12). Then place folded blankets or towels between the victim's ankles and thighs (not between the knees) and tie the legs together.

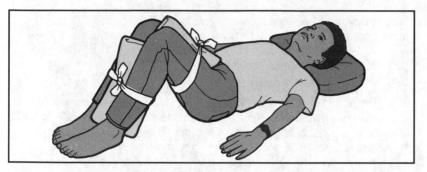

Figure 12
Immobilizing a knee that is already bent

Leg. Do not move a victim with an injured *upper leg* unless it is absolutely necessary. Wait for medical help to arrive. If you *must move* the victim, splint the injured thigh as you would an injured hip (as shown in Figure 11).

To immobilize an injured *knee* or *lower leg*, you'll need 2 padded boards (Figure 13a). Place a long board on the outside of the injured leg extending from the hip to below the heel. Place a second board on the inside of the leg, extending from the groin to below the heel. Secure the splint in at least 4 places. If you have nothing rigid on hand, you can fashion a splint by rolling up a blanket and placing it between the victim's legs, then tying his or her legs together in at least 4 places (Figure 13b).

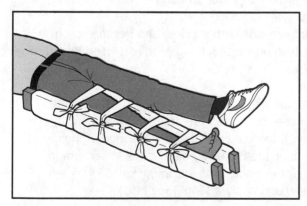
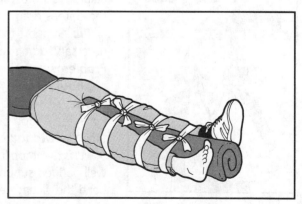

Figure 13 a, b
Two ways to immobilize a knee or lower leg

a

b

How to Apply a Splint

A splint is used to keep an injured body part from moving. This protects it from further damage until you have medical help. There are many commercially made splints, but you probably will have to improvise. Remember to check circulation after immobilizing the body part. Follow these general guidelines:

- Always care for wounds *before* applying a splint.
- Splint an injury in the position in which you found it. You will need strong supports to make a splint. Possibilities include boards, sticks, cardboard, ski poles, branches, broom handles, umbrellas, baseball bats, or rolled newspapers or magazines. If you have nothing rigid on hand, use a pillow or blanket. Sometimes you can tape an injured part of the body to an uninjured part to prevent movement.
- The splint must extend both above and below the injured area to keep it immobile.
- Secure the splint to uninjured parts of the body. Put ties or tape above and below, but not on top of, the injury.
- For ties, you can use cloth strips, neckties, torn sleeves, belts, etc.
- Make sure any knots are not pressing against the injury. Tie them securely, but not so tightly that circulation is impaired. If the area beyond the splint becomes pale, numb, or throbs with pain, loosen the ties. If an injured area swells after the splint has been applied, the splint could be too tight. Check often for swelling, and loosen the splint if necessary.

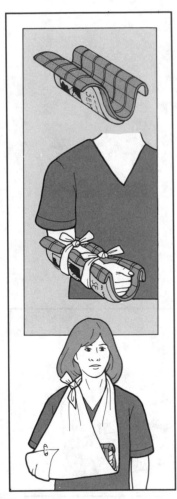

Figure 14
Immobilizing a wrist

Pelvis. Don't move a victim with an injured pelvis. Wait for medical help. If you must move the victim due to dangerous surroundings, use the clothes drag technique (see page 178).

Rib. Support the injured side with a pillow and get medical help. If necessary, administer first aid for breathing problems. (See **Breathing Problems** on page 79.)

Shoulder. See Arm.

Toe. Apply cold compresses and keep the injured foot elevated. Put some cotton between the injured toe and the toe next to it, and tape the two together. If the toe is misshapen, get medical help.

Wrist. Immobilize an injured wrist by placing the lower arm in a well-padded support (for example, a magazine) (Figure 14). Then bend the victim's elbow and apply a sling. (See box.)

How to Apply a Sling

A sling is a support made of cloth and tied around the neck. It is used to support shoulder, collarbone, and arm injuries. Sometimes you must splint an injury first, and then add a sling to support it. Always check the circulation of the limb after applying a splint and sling.

Triangular Sling

A sling can be made from a large triangular piece of cloth or, if necessary, from a sweater or pillow. For an adult, the base of the triangle should be about 55 inches long and the sides should be about 40 inches long. To apply a triangular sling, do the following:

1. Support the injured part and slide the sling under the arm on the victim's injured side. Pull the sling up past the victim's chin and over the shoulder of his or her uninjured side. The long side (base) of the triangle should be lined up along the victim's uninjured side; the point of the triangle opposite the base (apex) should lie under the elbow of the injured side (Figure 15a). Make sure there is enough extra cloth over the shoulder to tie a knot.
2. Pull the bottom corner over the victim's other shoulder. Leave the fingers showing (Figure 15b).
3. Tie the sling around the victim's neck, a little to one side so the knot does not press into the back of the neck (Figure 15c).
4. Fold over the extra cloth at the victim's elbow and secure it with safety pins (Figure 15d).
5. Check the sling for snugness; loosen if necessary.

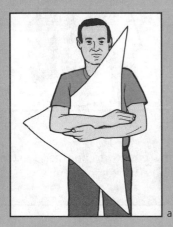
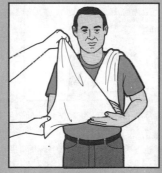
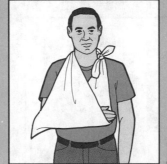
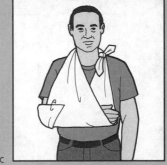

Figure 15 a, b, c, d
Applying a sling

(continued)

Improvised Sling

If you have no triangular cloth, you can fashion a sling from a shirt or sweater in much the same manner, tying the sleeves around the victim's neck (Figure 16).

Figure 16 a, b, c, d
Improvising a sling from a sweater

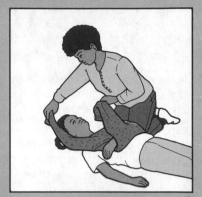

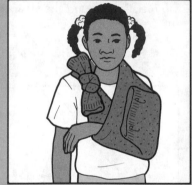

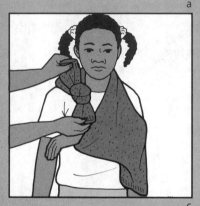

Chest Tie

Depending upon the specific injury, you may need to bind the sling to the body with another piece of cloth wrapped around the chest and tied on the uninjured side (Figure 17). This will prevent the injured arm from swinging away from the victim's body.

Figure 17 a, b
Binding a sling with a chest tie

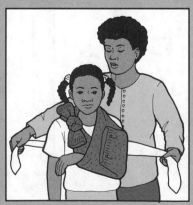

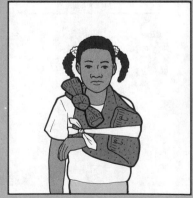

Breathing is basic to human life. All the cells of the human body need a constant supply of oxygen. Any problem that causes cells to receive less oxygen than they need is a medical emergency.

If you are to breathe properly, your brain, airway, lungs, ribs, and chest muscles must all be functioning correctly. Illness or injury can affect one or all of them.

As you inhale, muscles make your chest expand and suck air through your airway (nose, throat, and windpipe) into your lungs (Figure 18). In the lungs, oxygen enters the blood. The heart pumps freshly oxygenated blood from the lungs to the rest of the body.

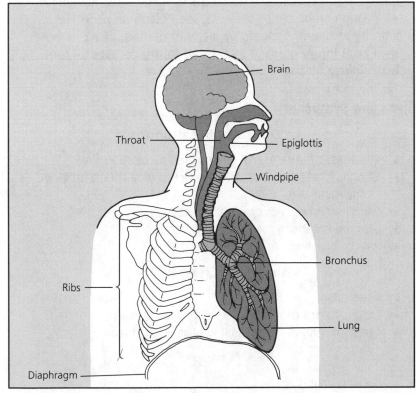

Figure 18
Anatomy of breathing

If difficulty breathing is accompanied by other signs of allergic reaction (including swelling of the face or tongue, hives, nausea, or flushed face), see **Allergic Reaction** on page 45.

If difficulty breathing is accompanied by other signs of an airway burn (including burns on the victim's face, singed nose hairs and eyebrows, or coughing), see **Burns** on page 84.

If the victim has stopped breathing (respiratory arrest), see **Cardiopulmonary Arrest** on page 89.

If you suspect the victim's airway is obstructed, see **Choking** on page 108.

If difficulty breathing is accompanied by other signs of drug overdose (including abnormal or inappropriate behavior, sweating, nausea, abnormal pupil size, or seizures), see **Drug Abuse** on page 124.

If difficulty breathing is accompanied by other signs of heart failure or heart attack (including chest pain, heavy perspiration, or heart palpitations), see **Heart Attack** on page 152.

If you suspect poisoning, or if difficulty breathing is accompanied by other signs of poisoning (including weakness, chills, abdominal pain, vision problems, or seizures), see **Poison** on page 163.

If difficulty breathing is caused by injury to the face, head, or nose, see **Facial Injury** on page 142, **Head Injury** on page 147, or **Nose Injury** on page 160.

Signs and Symptoms

Difficulty Breathing

- Shortness of breath; inability to breathe deeply
- Cough. (Can be wet or dry; the victim may cough up blood or frothy material.)
- Gurgling, wheezing, or whistling sounds
- Labored breathing; tense chest muscles
- Pale or bluish lips and fingernails

Airway or Chest Injury

- Chest pain
- Obvious signs of injury, such as bruises or open wounds
- Chest moving in an unusual way as victim breathes

Croup

- Barking cough
- Hoarseness
- Labored breathing

- Rapid breathing
- Chest pain
- Faintness; dizziness
- Numb fingers or toes

Difficulty Breathing

Difficulty breathing can be caused by injury, sudden illness, or ongoing medical problems (such as heart disease, emphysema, chronic bronchitis, or asthma). Shortness of breath associated with heart failure is due to fluid backing up into the lungs. Young, healthy people can suddenly become short of breath due to a collapse of a portion of their lung. High altitudes can also cause breathing problems.

- If the victim is having severe breathing problems, call EMS.
- If the victim is having chest pain with difficulty breathing, call EMS.
- If you can determine the cause of the victim's breathing problems (check for a medical ID tag), give first aid for that specific illness or injury.

DO NOT place the victim in a position he or she finds uncomfortable.

DO NOT place a pillow under the victim's head if he or she is lying down. This can close the airway.

DO NOT wait to see if the victim's condition improves before getting medical help. Get help now.

DO NOT give the victim anything by mouth.

1. Check the victim's ABCs. Open the airway; check breathing and circulation. If necessary, begin rescue breathing, CPR, or bleeding control. (See the Emergency Action Guides on pages 199–210.)

   If the victim is unconscious but breathing, try to determine whether he or she has a spinal injury. If spinal injury is possible, leave the victim in the position you found him or her. If spinal injury is not suspected, place the victim in the recovery position. (See page 183.)

   If the victim is conscious, allow him or her to get into a comfortable position. A conscious victim will naturally assume the position in which it is easiest to breathe. Remember to calm and reassure the victim, since breathing problems are extremely frightening. Anxiety can worsen the problem.

2. Loosen any constricting clothing.

3. Assist the victim with any medication he or she may have (for example, asthma inhaler or home oxygen).

4. Continue to monitor the victim's ABCs until you get medical help. *Do not* mistake drowsiness for an improvement in the victim's condition. *Do not* assume that the victim's condition is improving if you can no longer hear wheezing.

FIRST AID

Airway or Chest Injury

Direct trauma to the neck or chest can cause breathing problems. Internal injuries are often more severe than they look.

If the victim has a wound with an object stuck in it, don't remove the object. Instead, try to keep the object from being hit and get medical help immediately. (See **Wounds** on page 186.)

- If the victim's airway is injured or swelling, call EMS.
- If the victim's chest is injured, call EMS.

DO NOT move the victim unless it is absolutely necessary.
DO NOT give the victim anything by mouth.
DO NOT place the victim in a position he or she finds uncomfortable.
DO NOT place a pillow under the victim's head if he or she is lying down. This can close the airway.

1. Check the victim's ABCs. Open the airway; check breathing and circulation. If necessary, begin rescue breathing, CPR, or bleeding control. (See the Emergency Action Guides on pages 199–210.)

2. If there are no open wounds but the victim's chest moves in an uneven way as he or she breathes, suspect broken ribs. Firmly support the injured side.

3. If there are open wounds in the neck or chest, they must be closed immediately, especially if air bubbles appear in the wound. Bandage such wounds at once. (See **Wounds** on page 186.)

   A "sucking" chest wound allows air to enter the victim's chest cavity as he or she breathes; this can cause a collapsed lung. Bandage the wound with plastic wrap, a plastic bag, or gauze pads covered with petroleum jelly, sealing it except for one corner (Figure 19). This allows trapped air to escape from the chest but prevents air from entering the chest through the wound.

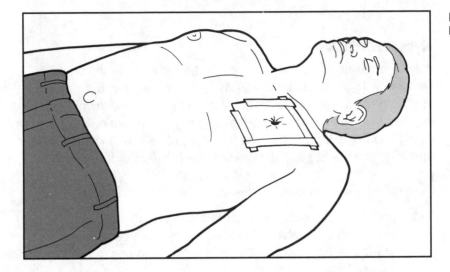

Figure 19
Bandaging a sucking chest wound

Croup

Croup usually affects young children and usually occurs at night. When croup occurs, be alert for epiglottitis, a life-threatening illness characterized by high fever, extreme difficulty breathing, and drooling.

- If the child is having severe breathing problems, call EMS.
- Treat the fever.

DO NOT place the child in a position he or she finds uncomfortable.

DO NOT place a pillow under the child's head if he or she is lying down. This can close the airway.

1. Calm and reassure the child. Anxiety makes breathing problems worse.

2. Take the child into the bathroom, close the door, and run the shower or bath full force, creating as much steam as possible (do not hold the child close to hot water). Have the child breathe moist air for 20 minutes.

FIRST AID

If you cannot use the bathroom method, take the child out-side into the cool night air.

3. If labored breathing continues, or if the child develops bluish lips or fingernails, get medical help. Do not mistake drowsiness for an improvement in the child's condition.

FIRST AID

Hyperventilation

Breathing too rapidly causes the carbon dioxide levels in the blood to fall quickly. Hyperventilation is usually caused by anxiety, but illness or injury can also be the cause. Asthma, head injury, fever, thyroid prob-lems, and certain medications can all cause hyperventilation. In the young and the elderly, one of the first signs of serious illness is rapid breathing. In infants, rapid breathing is the first sign of illness and precedes fever.

For rapid breathing due to anxiety:

1. Encourage the victim to breathe more slowly and to hold his or her breath after inhaling, *or* have the victim breathe in and out of a paper bag, *or* have the victim breathe in and out of cupped hands.

2. Calm and reassure the victim. Anxiety can cause hyperventila-tion, which can cause greater anxiety — a vicious cycle that needs to be stopped. Encourage the victim to talk and distract him or her to help break the cycle.

3. If the victim faints, normal breathing will resume. (See **Uncon-sciousness** on page 182.)

Burns

Burns can be caused by dry heat (for example, fire), wet heat (steam or hot liquids), radiation, friction, electricity, or chemicals. An *airway burn* affects any part of the airway (nose, throat, and windpipe) and can be caused by inhaling smoke, steam, superheated air, or toxic fumes, often in a poorly ventilated space.

The seriousness of a skin burn is determined by two major factors: the size of the burn and its depth. Before giving first aid, consider how extensively burned the victim is and try to determine the depth of the most serious part of the burn. Then treat the entire burn accordingly. Knowing how the burn occurred is helpful, since different sources cause different types of burns. If you are in doubt, treat it as a severe burn.

Giving immediate first aid before medical help is received may lessen the severity of the burn. Prompt medical attention to serious burns can help prevent scarring, disability, and deformity.

If the victim has received a chemical burn, see **Chemical Exposure** on page 97.

If the victim has been electrocuted, see **Electrical Injury** on page 132.

If the victim has burned his or her eye(s), see **Eye Injury** on page 136.

If the victim has an airway burn from inhaling smoke or chemicals, see **Poison** on page 163.

Signs and Symptoms

- Red skin
- Swelling
- Blisters
- Peeling skin
- White or charred skin
- Pain. (The victim's degree of pain is not related to the severity of the burn, since the most serious burns are painless.)
- Shock. (Watch for pale and clammy skin, weakness, bluish lips and fingernails, and decreasing alertness.)

Signs and symptoms of an airway burn include:

- Charred mouth; burned lips
- Singed nose hairs or eyebrows
- Burns on the head, face, or neck
- Difficulty breathing; coughing

Minor Burns

A burn that is both superficial (red skin and perhaps a blister) and smaller than a quarter can be treated as a minor burn.

- Check for other injuries. Administer first aid for more serious injuries first.

FIRST AID

DO NOT apply ointment, cream, oil, spray, or any household remedy. This can interfere with proper healing.

DO NOT allow the burn to become contaminated. Avoid breathing or coughing on the burn.

1. Cool the burn by immediately immersing it in cold water (not ice water) or putting it under gently running cold water for at least 10 minutes. A clean, cold, wet towel will also help reduce pain. *Do not* apply ice directly to the skin. For a minor mouth burn, give the victim ice to suck.

2. If a blister forms, leave it alone.

3. Pat the area dry with a clean (preferably sterile) cloth and cover the burn with a dry, sterile, nonadhesive dressing to help prevent contamination and infection. *Do not* use a fluffy (cotton) or adhesive dressing.

4. Protect the burn from pressure and friction.

5. Seek medical help for any burn that involves the airway, eyes, face, hands, or genitals.

More on the Subject

If the burn does not heal normally, get medical advice. If signs of infection develop—including increased pain, redness, swelling, discharge, swollen lymph nodes, or red streaks spreading from the burn toward the heart—get medical help immediately. Make sure the victim is up to date on tetanus immunizations.

FIRST AID

Superficial but Extensive Burns

Burns that are not deep but cover more than one part of the body require prompt medical attention.

- If the victim shows signs of shock, call EMS.
- If the victim has an airway burn, call EMS.

DO NOT disturb blisters or dead skin.

DO NOT apply ointment, cream, oil, spray, or any household remedy. This can interfere with proper healing.

DO NOT allow the burn to become contaminated. Avoid breathing or coughing on the burn.

1. Calm and reassure the victim. Burns can be extremely painful.

2. Remove clothing from the burned area *if* it comes off easily, but otherwise *do not* disturb the burn. Remove any rings or constricting items, since the burned area will swell.

3. If the burned area is smaller than the victim's chest, cool the burn by covering it with clean, cold, wet towels. Immediate cooling can help reduce the effects of the burn on deeper layers of skin. *Do not* apply ice directly to the skin.

   If the burn is larger than the victim's chest, *do not* use cold compresses and *do not* immerse the burn in cold water; there is a risk of overcooling the victim.

4. Cover the burn with a dry, sterile, nonadhesive dressing to help prevent contamination and infection. Plastic wrap can be used as a temporary dressing. *Do not* use a fluffy (cotton) or adhesive dressing.

5. If fingers or toes have been burned, separate them with dry, sterile, nonadhesive dressings.

6. Elevate the burned area and protect it from pressure and friction.

7. Take steps to prevent shock. Lay the victim flat, elevate his or her feet 8 to 12 inches, and cover the victim with a coat or blanket. *Do not* place the victim in the shock position if you suspect any head, neck, back, or leg injury or if the position makes the victim uncomfortable. (See **Shock** on page 172.)

8. Stay with the victim until you have medical help.

More on the Subject

Keep dressings clean and dry and change them as needed. If the burn does not improve, get medical help. If signs of infection develop — including increased pain, redness, swelling, discharge, swollen lymph nodes, or red streaks spreading from the burn toward the heart — get medical help immediately. Make sure the victim is up to date on tetanus immunizations.

FIRST AID

Severe Burns

Any deep burn, even one that does not cover more than one part of the body, requires immediate medical attention.

- Call EMS.

DO NOT give the victim anything by mouth.

DO NOT apply cold compresses and *do not* immerse a severe burn in cold water. This can cause shock.

DO NOT disturb blisters or remove dead skin.

DO NOT apply ointment, cream, oil, spray, or any household remedy. This can interfere with proper healing.

DO NOT allow the burn to become contaminated. Don't breathe or cough on the burn.

1. Check the victim's ABCs. Open the airway; check breathing and circulation. If necessary, begin rescue breathing, CPR, or bleeding control. (See the Emergency Action Guides on pages 199–210.)

2. Remove clothing from the burned area *if* it comes off easily, but otherwise *do not* disturb the burn.

3. If possible, cover the burn with a dry, sterile, nonadhesive dressing to help prevent contamination and infection. Plastic wrap can be used as a temporary dressing. *Do not* use a fluffy (cotton) or adhesive dressing.

4. If fingers or toes have been burned, separate them with dry, sterile, nonadhesive dressings.

5. Elevate the burned area and protect it from pressure and friction.

6. Take steps to prevent shock. Lay the victim flat, elevate his or her feet 8 to 12 inches, and cover the victim with a coat or blanket. *Do not* place the victim in the shock position if you suspect any head, neck, back, or leg injury or if the position makes the victim uncomfortable. (See **Shock** on page 172.)

7. Continue to monitor the victim's ABCs until you have medical help.

FIRST AID

Airway Burn

An airway burn can cause the airway to swell and can lead to suffocation. Signs of an airway burn may not appear for 24 hours.

- Remove the victim from a smoky or fume-filled area, or from any source of inhalation poisoning. (See page 167.)
- Call EMS.

DO NOT place a pillow under the victim's head if he or she is lying down. This can close the airway.

1. Calm and reassure the victim.

2. A conscious victim will naturally assume the position in which it is easiest to breathe. If the victim is unconscious and you do not suspect spinal injury, place him or her in the recovery position. (See page 183.)

3. Stay with the victim until you have medical help.

Cardiopulmonary Arrest

Cardiopulmonary arrest is a combination of two life-threatening conditions: *respiratory arrest* (no breathing) and *cardiac arrest* (no heartbeat).

Cardiopulmonary resuscitation, or CPR, keeps the body's cells supplied with oxygen until normal body functions resume. CPR is a combination of *rescue breathing* (which provides oxygen to the victim's lungs) and *chest compressions* (which keep the victim's heart circulating oxygenated blood). All the body's cells need a steady supply of oxygen, especially the brain cells, which can start to die after 4 to 6 minutes without it.

Before performing CPR, you must check the victim's ABCs and determine that the victim is not breathing *and* has no pulse. Chest compressions should never be performed unless there is no pulse — that is, the victim's heart is not beating.

CPR can be lifesaving, but it is best performed by those who have been trained in a CPR course.

If you are alone with a victim of cardiopulmonary arrest, it's important to shout for help and try to have someone call EMS while you attend to the victim. When you are trained in CPR, you will probably learn that if you are unable to get help, you should perform CPR for 1 minute and then call EMS. However, if you are unsure about how to proceed, call EMS.

If You Suspect a Head, Neck, or Back Injury

If you think the victim might have a head, neck, or back injury, you will have to take that into account as you open the airway. Simply lift the chin rather than tilt the head back. If you cannot breathe air into the victim, then try tilting the head back very slightly.

Cardiopulmonary Arrest   89

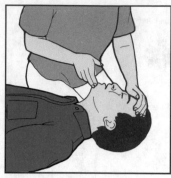
Figure 20
Head tilt/chin lift

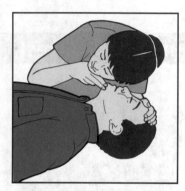
Figure 21
Look, listen, and feel for breathing

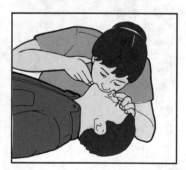
Figure 22
Give 2 breaths

Rescue breathing must be modified if you suspect a neck or back injury. See box on page 89.

Also keep in mind that the more quickly a victim of cardiopulmonary arrest receives medical care, the greater the chances of survival.

Signs and Symptoms

- Unconsciousness
- No breathing
- No pulse

CPR: Adult or Older Child (Over Age 8)

1. Check for consciousness: tap or gently shake the victim. Shout, "Are you OK?"

2. If there's no response, shout for help.

3. Position the victim: roll the victim onto his or her back, preferably on a firm surface with the head at the level of the heart. (Roll the victim as a unit, supporting the head and neck.) Straighten the victim's legs.

4. Kneel next to the victim, midway between the victim's chest and head.

5. Check the victim's ABCs:
   A. *Open the airway.* Use the head tilt/chin lift — place one hand on the victim's forehead. Then place two fingers of your other hand under the bony part of the victim's chin. Push on the forehead and lift the chin to tilt the head back (Figure 20).
   B. *Check breathing.* Look, listen, and feel for breathing for 3 to 5 seconds (Figure 21). (Put your ear to the victim's mouth. Chest movement alone may not mean breathing.) If the victim isn't breathing, give the victim 2 full breaths: pinch the nose shut and seal your lips tightly around the mouth (Figure 22). Give 2 breaths that last 1 to 1½ seconds. Watch for the victim's chest to rise with each breath. Let it fall before you give another breath.

      If you don't see the chest rise, retilt the victim's head and try again. If the victim's chest still doesn't rise, the airway is blocked. Begin first aid for an unconscious adult whose airway is blocked (page 110).

C. *Check circulation.* Use one hand to keep the victim's head tilted. With your other hand, check the carotid pulse on the victim's neck, on the side nearest you, for 5 to 10 seconds (Figure 23). (Place 2 fingers in the groove between the voice box and the muscle at the side of the neck to feel for a pulse. Don't use your thumb; you'll feel your own pulse.) Also check for and control any severe bleeding. (See **Bleeding** on page 62.)

6. Call EMS. Have someone else make the call if possible. Give the dispatcher a report on the victim's ABCs.

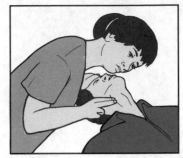

Figure 23
Check the pulse on the side of the neck

If the victim is now breathing and has a pulse, keep monitoring ABCs and give first aid for illness or injuries.

If the victim has a pulse but is not breathing, continue rescue breathing. Give 1 breath every 5 seconds. Listen for breathing. Recheck the pulse after every 12th breath (once a minute). Continue until EMS arrives, until someone else takes over, or until you are too exhausted to continue.

If the victim has no breathing and no pulse, begin CPR:

7. Position your hands: find the notch where the victim's ribs meet the sternum (breastbone) in the center of the chest. Place your middle finger on the notch and your index finger next to it. Then place the heel of your other hand next to and above your index finger, along the sternum (Figure 24, inset).

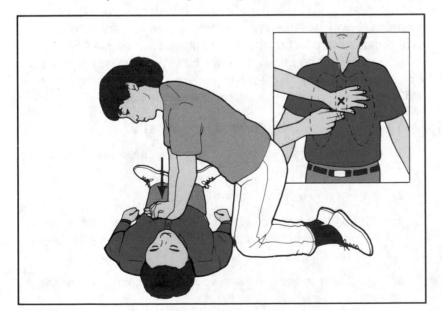

Figure 24
Position your hands and perform chest compressions

Remove your fingers from the notch and place the heel of this hand directly over the heel of your other hand. Keep your fingers off the victim's chest — hold them upward or interlace them.

8. Give 15 chest compressions: lean over the victim so your shoulders are over your hands. Lock your arms straight (Figure 24).

    Press down forcefully on the victim's sternum — use the weight of your body to depress the sternum 1½ to 2 inches. Release by lifting up, but don't remove your hands or let them shift. Give 15 chest compressions this way at the rate of 80 to 100 a minute. (Count aloud, "One and two and three and . . .")

    Don't rock back and forth — push straight down. Don't pause between compressions.

9. Open the airway with the head tilt/chin lift. Give 2 more breaths, watching for the chest to rise.

10. Continue to repeat this sequence of 15 compressions and 2 breaths for 4 cycles.

11. Recheck the pulse.

If the victim is breathing and has a pulse, stop performing CPR. Monitor the ABCs and give first aid for the illness or injuries.

If the victim has a pulse but is not breathing, continue rescue breathing. Give 1 breath every 5 seconds. Listen for breathing and recheck pulse every 12 breaths. If the pulse stops, resume CPR.

If the victim has no pulse and is not breathing, repeat the cycles of 2 breaths followed by 15 chest compressions until the victim revives, until help arrives, or until you are unable to continue.

CPR: Child (Age 1 to 8)

1. Check for consciousness: tap or gently shake the child. Shout, "Are you OK?"

2. If there's no response, shout for help.

3. Position the child: roll the child onto his or her back, preferably on a firm surface with the head at the level of the heart. (Roll the child as a unit, supporting the head and neck.)

4. Kneel next to the child with your knees against the child's side.

5. Check the child's ABCs:
   A. *Open the airway.* Use the head tilt/chin lift — place one hand on the child's forehead. Then place two fingers of your other hand under the bony part of the child's chin. Gently tilt the child's head back by pushing on the child's forehead and lifting the chin (Figure 25).
   B. *Check breathing.* Look, listen, and feel for breathing for 3 to 5 seconds (Figure 26). (Put your ear to the child's mouth. Chest movement alone may not mean breathing.) If the child isn't breathing, give the child 2 full breaths: pinch the nose shut and seal your lips tightly around the mouth. Give 2 breaths that last 1 to 1½ seconds (Figure 27). Watch for the child's chest to rise and fall with each breath. Let it fall before you give another breath.

      If you don't see the chest rise, gently retilt the child's head and try again. If the child's chest still doesn't rise, the child's airway is blocked. Begin first aid for an unconscious child whose airway is blocked (page 110).
   C. *Check circulation.* Use one hand to keep the child's head tilted. With your other hand, check the carotid pulse on the child's neck, on the side nearest you, for 5 to 10 seconds (Figure 28). (Place 2 fingers in the groove between the voice box and the muscle at the side of the neck to feel for a pulse. Don't use your thumb; you'll feel your own pulse.) Also check for and control any severe bleeding. (See **Bleeding** on page 62.)

6. Call EMS. Have someone else make the call if possible. Give the dispatcher a report on the child's ABCs.

If the child is now breathing and has a pulse, keep monitoring ABCs and give first aid for illness or injuries.

If the child has a pulse but is not breathing, continue rescue breathing. Give 1 breath every 4 seconds. Listen for breathing. Recheck the pulse after every 15th breath (once a minute). Continue until EMS arrives, until someone else takes over, or until you are too exhausted to continue.

If the child has no breathing and no pulse, begin CPR:

7. Position your hands: use the hand nearer the head to keep the child's head tilted. With the other hand, find the notch where the child's ribs meet the sternum (breastbone) in the center of the chest. Place your middle finger on the notch and your index finger next to it. Look where you put your

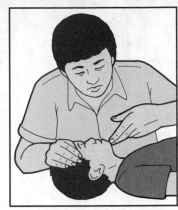
Figure 25 Head tilt/chin lift

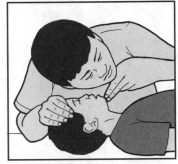
Figure 26
Look, listen, and feel for breathing

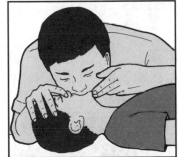
Figure 27 Give 2 breaths

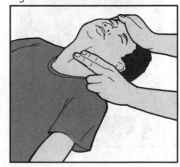
Figure 28
Check pulse on side of neck

Cardiopulmonary Arrest   93

Figure 29
Position your hands and
perform chest compressions

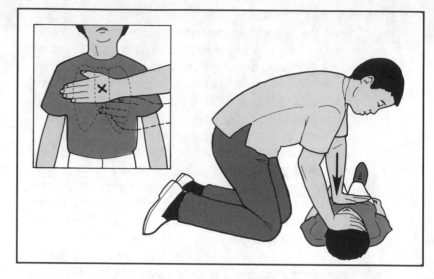

index finger. Now lift your hand and place the heel of your hand on the child's sternum, just above where your index finger was (Figure 29, inset). Keep your fingers off the child's chest — don't press on the ribs.

8. Give 5 chest compressions: with one hand, keep the child's head tilted. Lean over the child until your shoulder is right over your other hand and lock your arm straight (Figure 29).

   Press straight down on the child's sternum. Depress the sternum 1 to 1½ inches. Release by lifting up, but don't remove your hand or let it shift. Give 5 chest compressions this way at the rate of 80 to 100 a minute. (Count aloud, "One and two and three and . . .")

   Don't rock back and forth — push straight down. Don't pause between compressions.

9. Give the child 1 breath, watching for the chest to rise.

10. Continue to repeat this sequence of 5 compressions and 1 breath for 10 cycles.

11. Recheck the pulse.

If the child is breathing and has a pulse, stop performing CPR. Monitor the ABCs and give first aid for the illness or injuries.

If the child has a pulse but is not breathing, continue rescue breathing. Give 1 breath every 4 seconds. Listen for breathing and recheck pulse every 15 breaths (about once a minute). If the pulse stops, resume CPR.

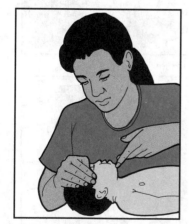

Figure 30
Head tilt/chin lift

94   **Part 2: First Aid**

If the child has no pulse and is not breathing, repeat the cycles of 1 breath followed by 5 chest compressions until the child revives, until help arrives, or until you are unable to continue.

CPR: Infant (Birth to Age 1)

1. Check for consciousness: tap or gently shake the baby's shoulder. See if the baby moves or makes a noise.
2. If no response, shout for help.
3. Position the baby. Roll the baby onto his or her back on a firm surface with the head at the level of the heart. (Roll the baby as a unit, supporting the head and neck.)
4. Check the baby's ABCs:

   A. *Open the airway.* Use the head tilt/chin lift — place one hand on the baby's forehead. Then place one finger (not your thumb) of your other hand under the bony part of the baby's chin. Tilt the baby's head back into a resting position by gently pushing on the baby's forehead and lifting the chin (Figure 30). Don't press on the soft tissue under the chin, and don't close the baby's mouth.

   B. *Check breathing.* Look, listen, and feel for breathing for 3 to 5 seconds (Figure 31). (Put your ear to the baby's mouth. Chest movement alone may not mean breathing.) If the baby isn't breathing, give the baby 2 breaths: keep the baby's head tilted with one hand and the baby's chin lifted with the other hand. Tightly seal your lips around the baby's mouth and nose. Give 2 full breaths that last 1 to 1½ seconds (Figure 32). Breathe forcefully, but not so hard that air goes into the baby's stomach. Watch for the baby's chest to rise with each breath. Let it fall before you give another breath.

   If you don't see the chest rise, gently retilt the baby's head and try again. If the baby's chest still doesn't rise, the baby's airway is blocked. Begin first aid for an unconscious baby whose airway is blocked (page 115).

   C. *Check circulation.* Use one hand to keep the baby's head tilted. With your other hand, check the brachial pulse in the baby's upper arm for 5 to 10 seconds (Figure 33). (Press gently with 2 fingers on the inside of the arm nearest you, between the elbow and the shoulder. Don't use your thumb; you'll feel your own pulse. If no pulse, put your ear close to the baby's chest and listen for a heartbeat.) Also check for and control any severe bleeding. (See **Bleeding** on page 62.)

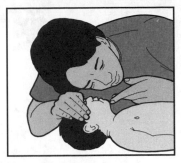
Figure 31
Look, listen, and feel for breathing

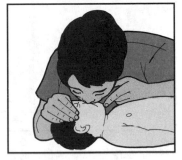
Figure 32
Give 2 breaths

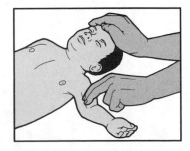
Figure 33
Check the pulse in the upper arm

Cardiopulmonary Arrest   95

5. Call EMS. Have someone else make the call if possible. Give the dispatcher a report on the baby's ABCs.

If the baby is now breathing and has a pulse, keep monitoring ABCs and give first aid for illness or injuries.

If the baby has a pulse but is not breathing, continue rescue breathing. Give 1 breath every 3 seconds. Listen for breathing. Recheck the pulse after every 20 breaths (once a minute). Continue until EMS arrives, until someone else takes over, or until you are too exhausted to continue.

If the baby has no breathing and no pulse, begin CPR:

6. Position your hands: use the hand nearer the head to keep the baby's head tilted. Now locate the baby's nipples and imagine a line running across the baby's chest between them. Put your index finger on the baby's sternum (breastbone) just below this line.

    Lay your next 2 fingers next to your index finger further down the baby's sternum. Now raise your index finger. Use only your 2 middle fingers to give chest compressions (Figure 34).

7. Give 5 chest compressions: with one hand, keep the baby's head tilted. Bend the elbow of your other arm.

    Press straight down on the baby's sternum with 2 fingers. Depress the sternum ½ to 1 inch. Release by lifting up, but don't remove your fingers or let them shift. Give 5 chest compressions this way at the rate of 100 a minute, or 5 compressions every 3 seconds. (Count aloud quickly, "One, two, three, four, five . . .")

    Don't rock back and forth — push straight down. Don't pause between compressions.

8. Give the baby 1 breath, watching for the chest to rise.

9. Continue to repeat this sequence of 5 compressions and 1 breath for 10 cycles.

10. Recheck the pulse.

If the baby is breathing and has a pulse, stop performing CPR. Monitor the ABCs and give first aid for the illness or injuries.

If the baby has a pulse but is not breathing, continue rescue breathing. Give 1 breath every 3 seconds. Listen for breathing and recheck pulse every 20 breaths (about once a minute). If the pulse stops, resume CPR.

If the baby has no pulse and is not breathing, repeat the cycles of 1 breath followed by 5 chest compressions until the baby revives, until help arrives, or until you are unable to continue.

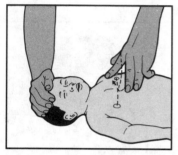

Figure 34
Position your fingers and perform chest compressions

If your skin comes in contact with chemicals, you may have a local reaction on the skin, a systemic (generalized body) reaction, or both. The effects of chemical exposure may be immediate or may develop over time — it depends on the chemical and the type of exposure. In general, very young people and older people, especially those with ongoing medical problems, have more severe reactions.

Chemical exposure is not always obvious. Suspect chemical exposure if an otherwise healthy person becomes ill for no apparent reason, particularly if you find an empty chemical container nearby.

When your skin reacts immediately to a chemical, quick first aid before you get medical help may greatly diminish the harmful effects of chemical exposure.

Many household products are made of harsh chemicals. It's important to read and follow label instructions, including any precautions. But you should know that the first aid procedure on the container may be either inaccurate or out of date.

Your local Poison Control Center is your best source of information.

If the victim has gotten chemicals into his or her eye(s), see **Eye Injury** on page 136.
If the victim has injected a drug, see **Drug Abuse** on page 124.
If the victim has swallowed or inhaled a dangerous chemical, see **Poison** on page 163.

Signs and Symptoms

- Rash, burns, or blisters on the skin
- Local pain despite little evidence of skin damage
- Bluish or bright red lips and skin
- Headache
- Dizziness
- Irritability
- Difficulty breathing
- Abdominal pain or generalized pains
- Seizures
- Unconsciousness
- Allergic reaction. (Signs and symptoms include dizziness; weakness; nausea; vomiting; difficulty breathing or swallowing; a flushed, swollen face or swollen tongue; hives; or itching.)

FIRST AID

Local Reaction
(Chemical Burns to the Skin)

- Try to identify the chemical or product involved.
- Call your local Poison Control Center for advice.

DO NOT become contaminated by the chemical as you give first aid.

DO NOT try to neutralize any chemical without consulting your local Poison Control Center or a physician.

DO NOT disturb blisters or remove dead skin from a chemical burn.

DO NOT apply any household remedy such as an ointment or salve to a chemical burn.

1. Quickly remove the chemical from the victim, taking care not to come into contact with it yourself. If the chemical is dry, brush off any excess with a towel. (Be careful not to brush it into your eyes.) Remove any contaminated clothing or jewelry.

2. Immediately drench the affected area with water. Keep flushing it with large quantities of fresh water for at least 15 minutes.

3. Apply cool, wet compresses to relieve pain.

4. Cover burns with loose, dry, sterile dressings. Protect the burned area from pressure and friction.

5. Get medical help. Don't leave the victim alone. Watch carefully for systemic reactions (see next section) until you have medical help.

FIRST AID

Systemic (Toxic) Reaction

- Remove the victim from the chemical.
- If the victim is having difficulty breathing, is having seizures, or is unconscious, call EMS.
- Try to identify the chemical or product involved.

1. Check the victim's ABCs. Open the airway; check breathing and circulation. If necessary, begin rescue breathing, CPR, or bleeding control. (See the Emergency Action Guides on pages 199–210 .)

   If the victim is unconscious but breathing, give first aid for unconsciousness. (See **Unconsciousness** on page 182.)

If the victim is conscious but having difficulty breathing, have the victim lie down. Give first aid for difficulty breathing. (See **Breathing Problems** on page 79.)

2. If the victim starts having seizures, protect him or her from injury and give first aid for convulsions. (See **Seizures** on page 168.)

3. Watch for a possible allergic reaction. (See **Allergic Reaction** on page 45.)

4. Take steps to prevent shock. Lay the victim flat, elevate his or her feet 8 to 12 inches, and cover the victim with a coat or blanket. *Do not* place the victim in the shock position if you suspect any head, neck, back, or leg injury; if he or she is having breathing problems; or if the position causes the victim discomfort. (See **Shock** on page 172.)

5. Continue to monitor the victim's ABCs until you get medical help. Don't leave the victim alone.

More on the Subject

Some people are exposed to potentially hazardous chemicals daily, either around the house or at work. The toxic effects of this kind of chemical exposure are cumulative. Low-level exposure over a prolonged period will cause changing symptoms as the chemical builds up in the victim's body.

Chest Injury   *See Breathing Problems*
Chest Pain   *See Heart Attack*

Childbirth

The following information is provided only for the rare occasion when delivery occurs unexpectedly and you cannot get medical help in time.

During childbirth, the contractions of the uterus dilate (open) the cervix and help the mother as she pushes the baby down the vagina (birth canal) and out the vaginal opening. Usually the baby is born

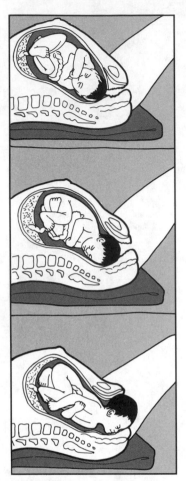

head first, facing down (Figure 35). After the baby is delivered, the placenta (afterbirth) detaches from the uterus and is also expelled.

The early stages of labor can last many hours. During this time, the cervix expands and the baby begins to move down the birth canal. Once the mother is actively pushing out the baby, delivery proceeds quickly.

Everyone should make arrangements for medical supervision during childbirth.

Signs and Symptoms

The following signs and symptoms suggest that delivery is not far off:

- Regular contractions that are less than 2 minutes apart (timed from the beginning of one contraction to the beginning of the next)
- Urge to have a bowel movement (due to pressure from the baby's head against the rectum)
- Strong urge to push; mother pushing and straining
- Bulging vaginal opening; baby's head visible during contractions. (It will recede, or pull back, between contractions.)
- Mother saying, ''The baby is coming!''

Rapid delivery is most common in women who have given birth quickly before, women who have given birth several times before, and women who go into labor prematurely. Premature delivery can be brought on by illness or injury. Rupture of the amniotic sac (''bag of waters'') usually indicates that the baby will be coming soon.

Figure 35
The baby moves through the birth canal

- If you are going to try to reach the nearest hospital, bring emergency childbirth supplies (see box on page 102) in the car.
- If there is no time to get to a hospital, first call EMS. Then get your emergency childbirth supplies (see box on page 102) and help the mother deliver the baby.
- If possible, get someone to help you.
- Keep everything as clean as possible before, during, and after delivery. Wear clean clothes and sterile rubber gloves. Choose the cleanest supplies you can find. Discard towels and bedding as soon as they become soiled.
- Watch for complications. (See box on page 106.)
- Remember that during childbirth, your concern is the well-being of 2 people.

DO NOT try to delay the delivery in any way. Crossing or holding the mother's legs, or pushing the baby's head back into the vagina, can seriously injure the baby.

DO NOT allow the mother to go to the toilet. Reassure her that the sensation of having to have a bowel movement means the baby is coming.

DO NOT pull the baby from the vagina.

DO NOT pull on the umbilical cord.

DO NOT cut the umbilical cord unless told to do so by medical personnel.

DO NOT let anyone cough or sneeze on mother or baby. Keep people with colds, unwashed hands, or open cuts at a distance.

DO NOT use chemicals or antiseptic products around mother or baby. Soap and clean water are best.

1. Calm and reassure the mother.

2. Remove all jewelry, including your watch. Wash your hands thoroughly with soap and water. Scrub under your fingernails. If possible, let your hands air dry. Wear sterile rubber gloves if possible.

3. Prepare a birthing area. Choose a large, flat surface such as a bed or table. It should be in a warm location that has good light. Put down a plastic sheet and cover it with a clean sheet, clean towels, or dry newspapers.

4. Make the mother as comfortable as possible. Have her remove any uncomfortable clothing. If she wants to lie on her

Emergency Childbirth Supplies

It's important to prepare the following supplies ahead of time. Take them with you if you will be traveling to a location where you may not be able to get medical care quickly (not advisable in the late stages of pregnancy). If you are taken completely by surprise, do the best you can to assemble the following:

- A flashlight (if the birthing area is not well lit)
- Pillows (to support the mother during delivery)
- A plastic sheet or plastic bags (to put under the mother)
- A clean sheet, clean towels, or fresh newspapers (to put on top of the plastic sheet)
- Clean, dry towels (at least three)
- Suction bulb
- Sanitary napkins
- Sterile gauze dressings
- Sterile rubber gloves
- Container (such as a plastic bag) for the placenta
- Container for soiled linens
- Receiving blankets for the baby
- Diaper

Since it may be necessary to cut the umbilical cord, you should also have on hand:

- Clean scissors. If you are preparing your supplies ahead of time, boil the scissors or soak them in rubbing alcohol for 20 minutes. If you are taken by surprise, wash the scissors with soapy water and rinse them off. A new single-edged razor blade is an alternative.
- Two clean cord ties, such as new white shoelaces or thick string. If you are preparing these ahead, boil them for 20 minutes, let dry, and wrap them up until needed. Do not use thread; it is too thin and will cut through the umbilical cord.

back, support her head and upper back with pillows. She should bend her knees and spread them wide apart. Alternative positions include squatting or lying on one side with one leg elevated.

5. Encourage the mother to take deep, slow breaths, especially during contractions.

6. If the mother has a bowel movement, wipe her from front to back (away from the vagina).

7. When you can see the baby's head (usually the back of the head shows first), place your hand against the perineum (the area below the vaginal opening) and apply gentle pressure during each contraction, asking the mother to push. This will help prevent the baby from coming too fast and tearing the mother's perineum.

   If something other than the baby's head shows first — for example, a buttock, foot, or hand — the baby is in an unusual position and the chances of a safe birth are reduced. Follow the steps for breech birth on page 107.

8. As the baby's head is delivered, support it with your hands (Figure 36a). It will naturally turn to one side. Clean the baby's mouth and nose with a dry towel. If you have a suction bulb, use that instead.

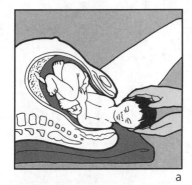
a

9. If the umbilical cord is wrapped around the baby's neck during delivery, hook it with your forefinger and gently but quickly slip it over the baby's head.

10. After the head is delivered, the rest of the baby's body usually follows quickly. Support the baby's head and shoulders as the baby emerges (Figure 36b). Remember, the baby will be slippery! It may help to hold on with a towel.

    If the baby's shoulder seems stuck, tell the mother to push hard. Press with your hands in the area just above the mother's pubic hair. You can also try lifting the mother's legs back toward her chest, keeping her knees bent and apart.

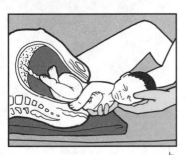
b

Figure 36a,b
Supporting the baby's head and shoulders

11. When the baby has been delivered, hold the baby face down, with the feet higher than the head, so that fluids can drain (Figure 37). If you have a suction bulb, gently suction out the nostrils and mouth. After the baby starts to cry, wipe the baby's nose and mouth again with a clean cloth. The baby may be blue, but will turn pink within minutes if he or she is breathing well.

    If the baby is not breathing, place the baby's head lower than the feet and tap the soles of the feet. Quickly stimulate the baby by gently rubbing the back. If the baby does not start breathing immediately, give 2 quick breaths. (See the Emergency Action Guides on pages 199–210.) After the baby starts breathing, resume the steps below.

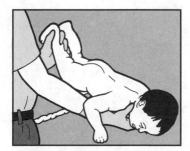

Figure 37
Allowing fluids to drain

12. *If the baby is breathing or crying*, dry the baby off. Then wrap the baby in dry towels, covering the head (not the face) to keep him or her warm. *Do not* wash off the baby or wash the face. Place the baby on the mother's chest (but be sure there is no tension on the umbilical cord). Encourage the baby to nurse; this will stimulate the mother to have the uterine contractions she needs to expel the placenta ("after-birth").

13. Tie a clean shoelace or clean, thick string around the umbilical cord about 4 inches (not closer) from the baby's navel. *Do not* use thread; it will cut through the cord. *Do not* cut the cord or pull on it. Tying off the cord is necessary to prevent continued circulation of the baby's blood to the placenta.

14. The mother will continue to have contractions. When the placenta is expelled, wrap it up or put it in a plastic bag. Be sure it goes to the hospital with the mother and baby.

15. If the mother is bleeding outside the vagina from a perineal tear, apply direct pressure with a sterile gauze dressing, washcloth, or fresh sanitary napkin until bleeding stops.

16. After the mother expels the placenta, firmly massage her abdomen to stimulate uterine contractions. This will help control uterine bleeding. Continue to knead the abdomen at frequent intervals for the first two hours after birth. Sometimes the uterus relaxes so completely that all contractions stop; massage can help restore the contractions.

17. Clean up the mother with soap and water. Keep both mother and baby warm. Hypothermia can occur rapidly in newborns. If all is well, have the mother recline while she nurses the baby. It is important that both be taken to a hospital as soon as possible for examination.

How to Cut the Umbilical Cord

Under normal circumstances, there is no rush to cut the umbilical cord. Placing one tie around it and leaving it alone is better than cutting it with unclean instruments. The baby will not be harmed if left attached to the placenta as long as both mother and baby receive prompt medical help.

If you cannot get medical help, you will have to tie and cut the cord after the baby has been delivered:

- Tie one clean shoelace or clean, thick string around the cord about 4 inches (not closer) from the baby's navel. Knot it firmly.
- Tie another shoelace around the cord about 8 inches from the baby's navel and knot it securely.
- Make sure the cord is securely tied in both places. If it isn't, the baby may bleed to death when the cord is cut.
- Cut the cord between the knots with sterile scissors, a heated knife, or a fresh razor blade (Figure 38). The cord should bleed only briefly when it is cut.
- Protect the cut ends of the cord with a clean cloth or sterile dressing.

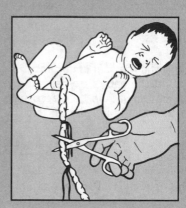

Figure 38
Cutting the umbilical cord after
it has been tied off

Possible Complications During Childbirth

Although they are rare, life-threatening complications can occur during childbirth. This is why it is important to call EMS when birth is about to take place outside a hospital setting.

Severe Bleeding

Excessive bleeding can occur for a variety of reasons before, during, or after delivery. Normal blood loss during childbirth is 1 to 2 cups. If the mother is hemorrhaging, she should be taken to the hospital immediately.

- Heavy painless bleeding or heavy bleeding before the baby is delivered may be an indication of *placenta previa*, a condition in which the placenta partially or completely blocks the cervix. Placenta previa is a medical emergency; the mother usually needs an immediate cesarean section.
- Heavy bleeding before delivery may be a sign of *placenta abruptio*, a condition in which the placenta begins to detach from the uterine wall too soon. Placenta abruptio also means that the mother requires an immediate cesarean section.
- Heavy bleeding during or after delivery may be a sign of *uterine rupture*, a condition in which the mother needs emergency surgery.

Meconium

Meconium (brown or greenish material that is the baby's first bowel movement) may appear as the baby is delivered. It can be a sign of fetal distress and can cause respiratory problems for the baby. Special equipment is needed to suction meconium out of a baby's airway. Immediate medical care is necessary.

Problems with the Umbilical Cord

- If the umbilical cord emerges from the birth canal before the baby, this is a medical emergency known as *cord prolapse*. With each contraction, the cord is squeezed and the baby's oxygen supply is interrupted. The mother needs an immediate cesarean section. The mother should be placed face down, buttocks up, with her knees into her chest, and immediately taken to the hospital in this position.
- If the umbilical cord *and* the baby's head appear at the perineum together and the mother cannot push the baby out with 1 or 2 contractions, the mother should be placed face down, buttocks up, with her knees into her chest and be taken to the hospital immediately in this position.
- If the umbilical cord is wrapped tightly around the baby's neck during delivery and you are unable to slip it over the baby's head, quickly tie off the cord in 2 places, then cut between the 2 ties (Figure 39). Do not cut the cord without tying it off first or the baby will bleed to death.

Second Baby

If a second baby appears in the birth canal, assist with this delivery as you did with the first. However, if the second baby's hand or shoulder comes before the head, an immediate cesarean section is probably required. Tie off the umbilical cord of the first baby (see page 104), then get the mother to the hospital immediately.

Problems with the Placenta

- If the placenta (afterbirth) is not expelled promptly (within half an hour), or if it does not all come out, there is a danger of hemorrhage. (*Do not* pull on the umbilical cord to get the placenta out.) The mother should be taken to a hospital immediately. Try having the baby nurse to stimulate uterine contractions.
- If the baby is delivered but the amniotic sac is still unbroken, tear the sac open with your fingers so the baby can breathe.

Breech Presentation

Most babies get into a head-down position in the uterus, but some do not. In a breech (head up) presentation, a buttock, foot, or knee may come out first. The danger with a breech is that although the baby's body may be easily delivered, there is a chance that the head — the largest part — may not follow.

- Allow the birth to proceed spontaneously.
- Have someone apply continuous, firm pressure to the area just above the mother's pubic hair.
- Support the baby's body as it is delivered.
- After the shoulders are delivered, check the time. Encourage the mother to push to deliver the head. If the head is not delivered within 3 minutes, raise the baby's body toward the ceiling until you can see his or her face (Figure 40). (*Do not* attempt to pull the baby from the vagina.) Wipe the baby's nose and mouth to clear the airway and wait for the rest of the head to be delivered. As long as the baby's face is free, there is no need to rush. Encourage the mother to keep pushing.

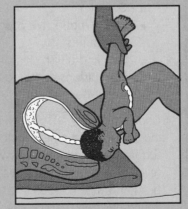

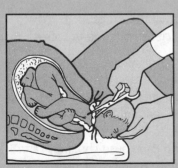

Figure 39
Cutting the umbilical cord from around the baby's neck after it has been tied off

Figure 40
Allowing a breech baby to breathe

Choking

Choking is your body's way of trying to remove a foreign object (such as food) from the airway.

A choking person's airway may be completely or partially blocked. A complete obstruction is life-threatening; a partial obstruction can be life-threatening if air exchange (the person's ability to breathe in and out) is or becomes poor. Treat any significant obstruction as a complete obstruction.

Without oxygen the brain can begin to die within 4 to 6 minutes. Rapid first aid for choking (abdominal thrusts, also called the Heimlich maneuver) can save a life.

If choking is accompanied by signs of allergic reaction (including swelling of the face or tongue, hives, nausea, or flushed face), see **Allergic Reaction** on page 45.

If the victim is a child who is having difficulty breathing, see **Breathing Problems** on page 79.

Signs and Symptoms

- Grabbing the throat with the hand (the universal distress signal for choking) (Figure 41)
- Gagging
- Weak, ineffective coughing; noisy breathing; high-pitched crowing sounds
- Pale and bluish skin, beginning with the face
- Convulsions and/or loss of consciousness (due to lack of oxygen)

Choking is often associated with eating (especially eating and laughing at the same time, eating with improperly fitted dentures, eating too fast, and failing to chew food well enough); alcohol consumption (even a small amount of alcohol affects awareness); trauma to the head and face (blood clots or bleeding can cause choking); and young children (particularly while eating, running, or playing with small objects). Suspect choking if you come upon an unconscious or convulsing person who recently may have been eating.

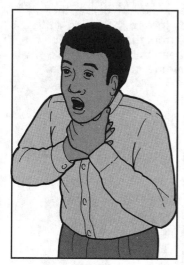

Figure 41
The universal distress signal for choking

Conscious Adult or Child
(Over 1 Year of Age)

- Ask the victim if he or she is choking. If the victim can't answer, the obstruction is life-threatening. Call EMS.
- Tell the victim you are going to try to help and ask for permission to proceed.

DO NOT interfere if the victim is coughing forcefully and has good air exchange (is able to breathe in and out). However, be ready to act instantly if the victim's air exchange worsens.

DO NOT pinch or poke an object that is lodged in the victim's throat. This might force it farther down the airway.

1. Perform abdominal thrusts as described below. (If you cannot get your arms around a large victim to give abdominal thrusts, or if the victim is noticeably pregnant, use chest thrusts — see box on page 112.)

2. Stand behind the victim.

3. Wrap your arms around the victim's waist.

4. Make a fist. Place the thumb side of your fist in the middle of the victim's abdomen, just above the navel and well below the lower tip of the breastbone (Figure 42, inset).

5. Grasp your fist with your other hand.

6. Keeping your elbows out, press your fist with a quick, upward thrust into the victim's abdomen (Figure 42). Each thrust is a separate attempt to clear the victim's airway by forcing air out the windpipe.

7. Continue performing this maneuver until the obstruction is cleared or the victim loses consciousness.

   If the victim loses consciousness, give first aid for an unconscious victim (see next section).

8. If the victim starts having seizures, see **Seizures** on page 168.

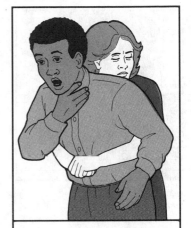
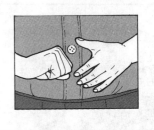

Figure 42
Performing abdominal thrusts
(Heimlich maneuver)

More on the Subject

Keep the victim still and get medical help. All choking victims should have a medical examination, since complications can arise not only from the incident but also from the first aid measures that were taken.

Occasionally, an object will enter the lung instead of being expelled. While the victim may appear to improve and breathe freely, a few days later the signs and symptoms of a foreign body in the lung will appear: wheezing, persistent cough, and pneumonia. Get medical help immediately.

FIRST AID

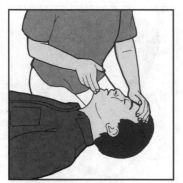

Figure 43
Head tilt/chin lift

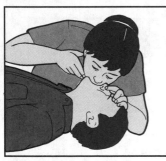

Figure 44
Give 2 breaths

Unconscious Adult or Child
(Over 1 Year)

- Call EMS

DO NOT pinch or poke an object that is lodged in the victim's airway. This might force it farther down the airway.

1. Place the victim on his or her back. Clear the victim's mouth if necessary; then check for breathing.
    If the victim is breathing, give first aid for unconsciousness. (See **Unconsciousness** on page 182.)
    If the victim is not breathing, your first priority is to give some air, if possible, and to try to restore the victim's breathing.

2. Begin rescue breathing. After tilting the victim's head back and lifting the chin (Figure 43), give 2 full breaths (Figure 44). Pinch the nose shut and seal your lips tightly around the mouth. Give 2 breaths that last 1 to 1½ seconds. Watch for the victim's chest to rise with each breath. Let it fall before you give another breath.

3. If the breaths will not go in, reposition the victim's head by tilting it further back and try again to give 2 full breaths.

4. If you are still unable to breathe into the victim, begin abdominal thrusts (see next step). If the victim is large or is noticeably pregnant, use chest thrusts (see box on page 112).

5. Straddle the victim's thighs.

6. Place the heel of one of your hands against the middle of the victim's abdomen, just above the navel and well below the lower tip of the breastbone.

7. Place your other hand on top of the first hand. Point your fingers toward the victim's head (Figure 45).

8. Give 6 to 10 quick thrusts, pressing your hands inward and upward. *Do not* press to either side. Each thrust is a separate attempt to clear the victim's airway by forcing air out through the windpipe.

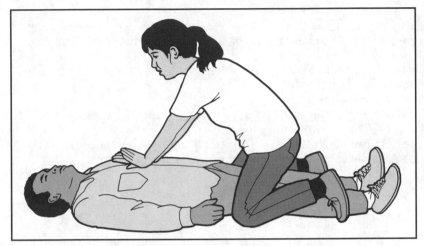

Figure 45
Performing abdominal thrusts
on an unconscious victim

If You Suspect a Head, Neck, or Back Injury

If you think the victim might have a head, neck, or back injury, you will have to take that into account as you open the airway. Simply lift the chin rather than tilt the head back. If you cannot breathe air into the victim, then try tilting the head back very slightly.

9. Check the victim's mouth. Do a finger sweep: grasp the victim's tongue and lower jaw between your thumb and fingers, and lift the jaw. Slide your index finger down the inside of the cheek to the base of the tongue.

    If the object has been dislodged, sweep it out with your index finger (Figure 46). Check to see if the victim is breathing. If breathing has not been restored, open the airway and give 2 more breaths.

    If the object has not been dislodged, try again to give 2 breaths. If the breaths will not go in, give another series of 6 to 10 thrusts, a check of the victim's mouth, and 2 full breaths.

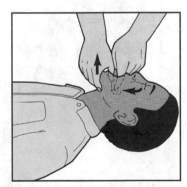

Figure 46
Sweep the object out

10. Continue this sequence of thrusts, checking the mouth, and breaths until the object is dislodged or you have medical help.

11. If the victim starts having seizures, see **Seizures** on page 168.

How to Perform Chest Thrusts for Large or Pregnant Victims

If the victim is large or is noticeably pregnant, use chest thrusts instead of abdominal thrusts.

Conscious Victim

1. Stand behind the choking victim (he or she can be standing or sitting). Place your arms under the victim's armpits.
2. Place the thumb side of one fist on the middle of the victim's breastbone (Figure 47). *Do not* place your fist on the ribs or at the lower tip of the breastbone.
3. Grasp your fist with your other hand.
4. Give quick, repeated thrusts, pushing your fist inward and upward. Each thrust is a separate attempt to clear the victim's airway by forcing air out the windpipe.
5. Continue performing this maneuver until the obstruction is cleared or the victim loses consciousness. If the victim loses consciousness, give first aid for an unconscious victim (see below).

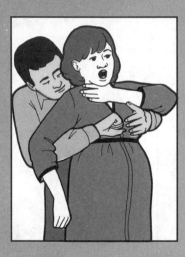

Figure 47
Doing chest thrusts on a pregnant
or large conscious victim

Unconscious Victim

1. Place the victim on his or her back on a firm, flat surface.
2. Kneel next to the victim's chest.
3. Place the heel of your hand in the middle of the victim's breastbone. *Do not* place your hand on the ribs or on the tip of the breastbone.
4. Place the heel of your other hand on top of your first hand. Keep your fingers off the victim's chest. Either hold your fingers upward or interlace them (Figure 48).
5. Give quick, repeated thrusts, pushing the heel of your hand downward, compressing the victim's chest 1½ to 2 inches. Each thrust is a separate attempt to clear the victim's airway by forcing air out the windpipe.

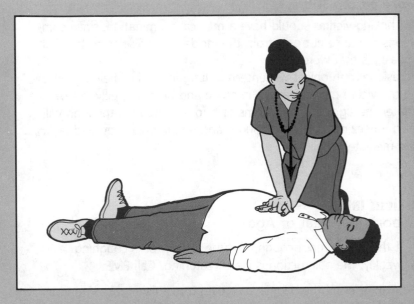

Figure 48
Doing chest thrusts on a pregnant
or large unconscious victim

6. Check the victim's mouth. Do a finger sweep: grasp the victim's tongue and lower jaw between your thumb and fingers, and lift the jaw. Slide your index finger down the inside of the cheek to the base of the tongue.

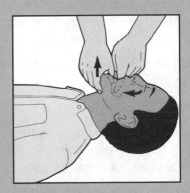

Figure 49
Sweep the object out

If the object has been dislodged, sweep it out with your index finger (Figure 49). Check to see if the victim is breathing. If breathing has not been restored, open the airway and give 2 more breaths.

If the object has not been dislodged, try again to give 2 breaths. If the breaths will not go in, give another series of 6 to 10 thrusts, a check of the victim's mouth, and 2 full breaths.

7. Continue this sequence of thrusts, checking the mouth, and breaths until the object is dislodged or you have medical help.
8. If the victim starts having seizures, see **Seizures** on page 168.

More on the Subject

All choking victims should have a medical examination, since complications can arise not only from the incident but also from the first aid measures that were taken.

Occasionally an object will enter the lung instead of being expelled. While the victim may appear to improve and breathe freely, a few days later the signs and symptoms of a foreign body in the lung will appear: wheezing, persistent cough, and pneumonia. Get medical help immediately.

FIRST AID

Conscious Infant
(Newborn to 1 Year of Age)

- If the baby cannot cough, breathe, or cry, or is coughing weakly, the obstruction is life-threatening. Call EMS.

DO NOT interfere if the baby is coughing forcefully and has good air exchange (the ability to breathe in and out). However, be ready to act instantly if air exchange worsens.

DO NOT pinch or poke an object that is lodged in the baby's airway. You might force it farther down the airway.

1. Give the baby back blows as follows. Place the baby face down along your forearm with the head lower than the rest of the body.

2. Support the baby's head with your hand, holding the jaw between your index finger and thumb.

3. Rest your forearm on your thigh.

4. Give 4 back blows with the heel of your hand, striking the infant's back forcefully between the shoulder blades (Figure 50). Each blow is a separate attempt to dislodge the object.

5. Immediately give the baby chest thrusts as follows. Turn the baby onto his or her back against your thigh or on a firm surface, with the baby's head lower than the chest.

6. Place your index finger and middle finger on the baby's breastbone just below the nipples (Figure 51).

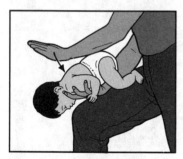

Figure 50
Performing back blows

7. Give 4 quick thrusts down, depressing the breast ½ to 1 inch each time. Each thrust is a separate attempt to clear the baby's airway by forcing air out through his or her windpipe.

8. Continue this series of 4 back blows and 4 chest thrusts until the object is dislodged or the baby loses consciousness. If the baby loses consciousness, give first aid for an unconscious infant (see next section).

9. If the baby starts having seizures, see **Seizures** on page 168.

More on the Subject

All choking victims should have a medical examination, since complications can arise not only from the incident but also from the first aid measures that were taken.

Occasionally an object will enter the lung instead of being expelled. While the victim may appear to improve and breathe normally, in a few days signs and symptoms of a foreign body in the lung will appear: wheezing, persistent cough, and pneumonia. Get medical help immediately.

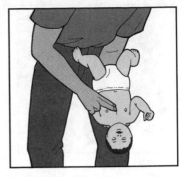

Figure 51
Performing chest thrusts

Unconscious Infant
(Newborn to 1 Year of Age)

- Call EMS.

DO NOT pinch or poke an object that is lodged in the baby's airway. This might force it farther down the airway.

1. Place the baby on his or her back.

2. *Open the airway.* Use the head-tilt/chin-lift—place one hand on the baby's forehead. Then place one finger (not your thumb) of your other hand under the bony part of the baby's chin. Tilt the baby's head back into a resting position by gently pushing on the baby's forehead and lifting the chin (Figure 52). Don't press on the soft tissue under the chin, and don't close the baby's mouth.

FIRST AID

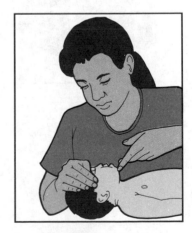

Figure 52
Head tilt/chin lift

Choking 115

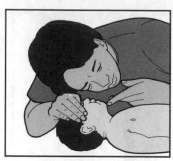

Figure 53
Look, listen, feel for breathing

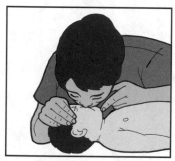

Figure 54
Give 2 breaths

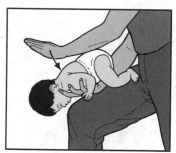

Figure 55
Performing back blows

3. *Check breathing.* Look, listen, and feel for breathing for 3 to 5 seconds (Figure 53). (Put your ear to the baby's mouth. Chest movement alone may not mean breathing.) If the baby isn't breathing, give the baby 2 breaths: keep the baby's head tilted with one hand and the baby's chin lifted with the other hand. Tightly seal your lips around the baby's mouth and nose. Give 2 full breaths that last 1 to 1½ seconds (Figure 54). Breathe forcefully, but not so hard that air goes into the baby's stomach. Watch for the baby's chest to rise with each breath. Let it fall before you give another breath.

4. If you are unable to breathe air into the baby, reposition the head by tilting it further back and again try 2 slow breaths.

5. If you are still unable to breathe air into the baby, give 4 back blows as follows. Place the baby face down along your forearm with the head lower than the rest of the body.

6. Support the baby's head with your hand, holding the jaw between your index finger and thumb.

7. Rest your forearm on your thigh.

8. Give 4 back blows with the heel of your hand, striking the infant's back forcefully between the shoulder blades (Figure 55). Each blow is a separate attempt to dislodge the object.

9. Immediately give the baby chest thrusts as follows. Turn the baby onto his or her back against your thigh or on a firm surface with the baby's head lower than his or her chest.

10. Place your index finger and middle finger on the baby's breastbone just below the nipples (Figure 56).

11. Give 4 quick thrusts down, depressing the breastbone ½ to 1 inch each time. Each thrust is a separate attempt to clear the baby's airway by forcing air out through his or her windpipe.

12. Grasp the baby's tongue and lower jaw between your thumb and fingers, and lift the jaw (Figure 57). Look into the mouth.
    If the object has been dislodged, sweep it out with your little finger. Check to see if the baby is breathing. If breathing has not been restored, continue rescue breathing.
    If the object has not been dislodged, give another 2 slow breaths, followed by 4 back blows and 4 chest thrusts, then check the baby's mouth again.

13. Continue this sequence of 2 slow breaths, 4 back blows, 4 chest thrusts, and checking the mouth until the object is dislodged or you get medical help.

14. If the baby starts having seizures, see **Seizures** on page 168.

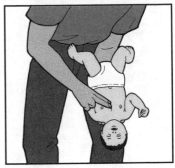

Figure 56
Performing chest thrusts

More on the Subject

All choking victims should have a medical examination, since complications can arise not only from the incident but also from the first aid measures that were taken.

Occasionally an object will enter the lung instead of being expelled. While the victim may appear to improve and breathe freely, a few days later the signs and symptoms of a foreign body in the lung may appear: wheezing, persistent cough, and pneumonia. Get medical help immediately.

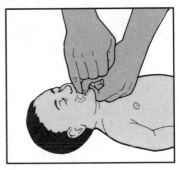

Figure 57
Sweep the object out

Cold Exposure

Exposure to cold can lead to both *frostbite* (in which your skin freezes) and *hypothermia* (in which your body's internal temperature drops below normal). Both conditions may start out with mild symptoms. But things can get worse quickly until the situation is life- or limb-threatening.

Frostbite occurs only outdoors in the cold. But hypothermia can occur indoors as well because many things can make your body lose heat.

Signs and Symptoms

Frostbite

- Mild frostbite: skin that is red and painful (early frostbite) or white and numb (tissue has started to freeze).
- Severe frostbite: blisters; gangrene (blackened tissue that died after blood vessels froze); hard, frozen skin (frostbite can penetrate all the way down to blood vessels and bone).

Factors that can contribute to frostbite include extreme cold; wet clothes; high winds ("wind chill"); and poor circulation, which can be caused by tight clothing or boots, cramped positions, fatigue, certain medications, smoking, drinking alcohol, or diseases that affect the blood vessels, such as diabetes. Frostbite is most common on extremities (fingers, toes, earlobes, nose) and exposed skin (cheeks).

Hypothermia

- Mild hypothermia: shivering; urge to urinate; loss of coordination; confusion; areas of the body that are usually warm (for example, the armpits) are cold.
- Severe hypothermia: victim no longer shivering; stumbling; muscle stiffness; desire to be left alone; irregular, slow heartbeat; drowsiness; weakness; confusion; slurred speech; difficulty seeing; uncooperative or irrational behavior. Signs and symptoms can progress to rigid muscles, unconsciousness, coma, and cardiac arrest.

Factors that contribute to hypothermia include extreme cold, wet clothes, being in cold water (assume that anyone pulled from cold water is hypothermic), and spending long periods in a cold environment or underheated room. Those who are most likely to have hypothermia are babies (newborns can rapidly become hypothermic); the elderly; people in poor health; or people with poor circulation because of certain medications, smoking, drinking alcohol, or diseases that affect the blood vessels, such as diabetes.

FIRST AID

Frostbite

- If the victim is mildly frostbitten, give first aid and get medical help as soon as possible.
- If the victim is more than mildly frostbitten, call EMS.
- If the victim has both frostbite and hypothermia, give first aid

for the hypothermia first (see First Aid: Hypothermia, next section).

DO NOT thaw out a frostbitten area if you cannot keep it thawed.
DO NOT use direct heat (radiator, campfire, heating pad, hair dryer, etc.) to rewarm a frostbitten area.
DO NOT disturb blisters on frostbitten skin.
DO NOT massage the frostbitten area.

1. Move the victim to a warmer place. Remove any constricting clothing or jewelry.

2. Rewarm the frostbitten area for at least 30 minutes. *To rewarm hands or feet*, place them in warm (not hot) water (100° to 105° Fahrenheit). Keep circulating the water to aid the rewarming process. *To rewarm other areas* that cannot be placed in water, apply warm (not hot) compresses.
   Burning pain, swelling, and color changes may occur during rewarming. Rewarming is complete when the skin is soft and sensation returns.

3. Apply dry, sterile dressings to the frostbitten areas. Put dressings between frostbitten fingers or toes.

4. Move thawed areas as little as possible.

5. Prevent refreezing by wrapping the rewarmed areas.

6. Stay with the victim until you have medical help.

More on the Subject

Discourage the victim from smoking or drinking alcohol. Both interfere with blood circulation.

Hypothermia

FIRST AID

- If the victim has mild hypothermia, give first aid and get medical help as soon as possible.
- If the victim is more than mildly hypothermic, call EMS.
- If the victim has both hypothermia and frostbite, give first aid for the hypothermia first.

DO NOT assume that someone found lying still in the cold is dead.
DO NOT use your own comfort to decide if an area is warm enough, since people respond differently to cold.

DO NOT attempt to rewarm a severely hypothermic person without medical advice.

DO NOT use direct heat (hot water, heating pad, heat lamp, etc.) to rewarm the victim.

1. Check the victim's ABCs. Open the airway; check breathing and circulation. If necessary, begin rescue breathing, CPR, or bleeding control. (See the Emergency Action Guides on pages 199–210.)

   If the victim is breathing at a rate of less than 6 breaths per minute, start rescue breathing. (See the Emergency Action Guides on pages 199–210.) *Do not* start chest compressions, since this can trigger cardiac arrest in a victim of hypothermia.

   If the victim is moving, has a pulse, and is breathing at a rate of more than 6 breaths per minute, do not interfere. Monitor the victim's ABCs while you give first aid for hypothermia.

2. Handle the victim gently. People with hypothermia are at risk for cardiac arrest.

3. Prevent the victim from becoming any colder. Find shelter, if necessary. Take off any wet or constricting clothes and replace them with dry clothing.

4. Rewarm the victim, remembering to cover the head and neck. Use a space blanket or aluminum foil, if available, to keep in body heat. If necessary, use your own body heat to aid the rewarming. Apply warm compresses to the neck, chest wall, and groin. If the victim is alert and can easily swallow, give warm, sweetened fluids (nonalcoholic) to aid in the rewarming process.

5. Stay with the victim until you have medical help.

More on the Subject

Discourage the victim from smoking or drinking alcohol. Both interfere with blood circulation. Hypothermia is one of the body's remarkable responses to cold and can actually be protective of the brain and heart.

Convulsions *See Seizures*

Diabetic Reaction *See Unconsciousness*

Dizziness *See Unconsciousness*

Drowning

Drowning can happen in many ways, but all deaths from drowning are due to lack of oxygen (asphyxiation). It's not important whether or not the lungs fill up with water, or whether the water is salt or fresh. What matters is how much oxygen continues to reach the victim's brain.

Water temperature makes a difference because your body responds in remarkable self-preserving ways to extreme cold. It's sometimes possible to revive a drowning victim even if that person has been in cold water (below 70° Fahrenheit) for a long period.

A person who is drowning usually cannot shout for help, so it's important to be alert for signs of a drowning emergency. Most drownings occur within a short distance of safety. Suspect an accident if you see someone in the water fully clothed. Watch for uneven swimming motions, which indicate a swimmer is tiring. Often the body sinks and only the head shows above water.

In a near-drowning emergency, immediate action and first aid can prevent a drowning death.

Signs and Symptoms

- Blueness of the face, especially the lips and ears
- Cold skin and pale appearance
- No breathing

Drowning can happen when a swimmer has muscle cramps in the legs or stomach; when there is a sudden illness (fainting, seizure, stroke, heart attack); in connection with boating accidents; and when there has been alcohol consumption (drinking when boating or swimming).

Drowning

- Call EMS.
- Rescue the drowning person if you can do so without endangering yourself. (See box on page 122.)

FIRST AID

How to Rescue a Drowning Person

When someone is drowning, get help right away, but do not place yourself in danger. Do not get into the water or onto the ice yourself unless there is no other alternative. Once you have reached the victim, offer reassurance and slowly pull him or her to safety. If back or neck injury is suspected (for example, in a diving accident), keep the victim's head and neck in line with the rest of his or her body. (See **Spinal Injury** on page 175.)

EMS should always be notified in a drowning emergency.

Water Rescue

Unless you are trained in water rescue, it is best not to swim to the aid of a drowning person. In desperation he or she may grab you and pull you under. Whenever possible, give the victim something to hold onto as you pull him or her to safety.

The four methods of water rescue are:

1. *Reaching Assist.* Extend your arm or leg or any long, rigid object, such as a pole or paddle, to the victim (Figure 58). If you have nothing rigid, use a towel.
2. *Throwing Assist.* Throw a flotation device, such as an inner tube, buoy, or life ring, to the victim (Figure 59). If your device has a rope attached, pull the victim to safety.
3. *Rowing Assist.* If a rowboat is available and you have the skills to use it, row out to the victim. Throw the victim a flotation device, or allow him or her to hang onto your oar or to the stern of the boat as you row to shore (Figure 60). If possible, pull the victim aboard over the rear of the boat (the stern). This will help prevent capsizing.
4. *Wading Assist.* Remove any heavy objects, but if the water is cold, leave your clothes on. Wade out to the victim, being aware of any strong currents. If possible, use a *reaching assist* and extend something to the victim for him or her to grab (Figure 61). Use a stick to test the depth of the water; you can also hold it out to the drowning person.

Ice Rescue

If someone has broken through the ice, find a secure place from which to help. Stay as far away from the break in the ice as possible. Stay off the ice altogether unless there is no alternative and there is a third rescuer on land. Use a *reaching assist* and extend a ladder or stick (Figures 62 and 63), or, if enough bystanders are present, forming a human chain of rescuers lying flat on the ice (Figure 64).

You can also use a *throwing assist* and throw the victim anything that will support him or her, preferably something with a line attached, such as an ice cross (Figure 65). Then, if possible, haul the victim over the ice to safety.

Keep in mind that victims who have fallen through the ice become hypothermic very rapidly and may not be able to grasp objects within their reach or hold on while being pulled to safety.

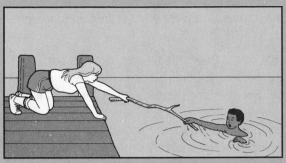

Figure 58   Reaching assist

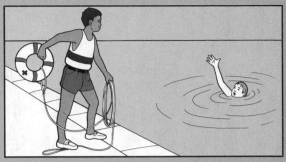

Figure 59   Throwing assist

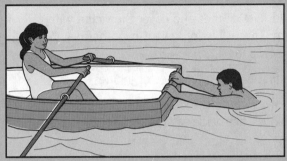

Figure 60   Rowing assist

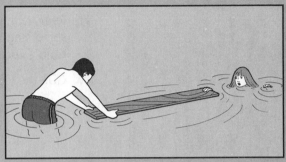

Figure 61   Wading assist

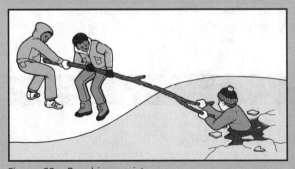

Figure 62   Reaching assist

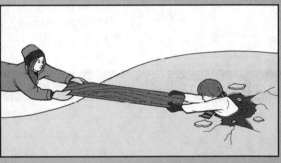

Figure 63   Alternative reaching assist

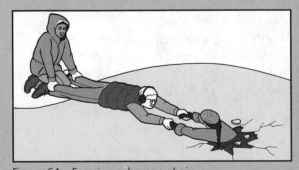

Figure 64   Forming a human chain

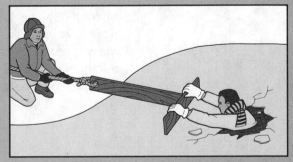

Figure 65   Throwing assist using an ice cross

DO NOT assume that a victim cannot or should not be helped.
DO NOT attempt a swimming rescue unless you are trained in water rescue.

1. Check the victim's ABCs. Open the airway; check breathing and circulation. If necessary, begin rescue breathing, CPR, or bleeding control. (See the Emergency Action Guides on pages 199–210.)

    If the ABCs are present and you do not suspect a spinal injury, place the victim in the recovery position. (See page 183.) This will keep the victim's airway clear if he or she vomits.

2. Remove any cold, wet clothes and cover the victim with something warm. This will help prevent hypothermia. (See **Cold Exposure** on page 117.)

3. Give the victim first aid for any illness or injuries.

4. As the victim revives, he or she may cough and experience difficulty breathing. Calm and reassure the victim until you get medical help.

More on the Subject

All near-drowning victims should be checked by a physician. Even though victims may revive quickly at the scene, lung complications are common.

Drug Abuse

A drug is any substance — including caffeine, nicotine, alcohol, a prescription medication, an over-the-counter medication, or an illegal preparation — that affects how the body functions. The effects of any particular drug depend upon the individual's body chemistry, the type of drug, how it is taken, and how much is taken.

Drug abuse is the misuse or overuse of a drug, including alcohol. Many street drugs have no therapeutic benefits; to use them at all is a form of drug abuse. Sometimes legitimate drugs are abused. For example, some people take more than the recommended dose of a prescribed medication or take a medication with alcohol or another drug.

Many drugs are physically or psychologically addictive. With some drugs, the addiction is gradual; with others, such as crack (see box on page 126), an addiction can happen almost immediately. Someone who has developed a *drug dependence* becomes obsessed with obtaining a drug and believes he or she cannot function normally without it. If a drug-dependent person tries to stop taking the drug, he or she may experience *withdrawal* symptoms. On the other hand, a user who continues to take the drug may develop a *drug tolerance* and need to take the drug in larger and larger quantities to get the same effect — until the dose is large enough to be potentially fatal. With some drugs, there's a fine line between getting high and getting killed. How much is too much is impossible to predict — it depends on the individual and, with street drugs, on the purity. A dose that is large enough to be toxic is called an *overdose*. Prompt medical attention may save the life of someone who accidentally or deliberately overdoses.

Besides overdose, the risks of drug abuse include poisoning, permanent brain or organ damage, death from careless injection, death from communicable diseases (such as AIDS and hepatitis), and fatal accidents due to impaired judgment and coordination.

Drug abuse tends to escalate from occasional to regular use. No one starts out with a drug problem. Signs and symptoms of prolonged drug use include personality changes, unreliable or extreme behavior, withdrawal from others, depression, changes in sleeping or eating habits, listlessness or restlessness, red eyes, constant sniffing, and needle marks. If someone you know is abusing drugs, get professional help immediately. Many individuals, organizations, and hotlines are there to help you. (See Resources at the back of this book.)

Drug emergencies are not always easy to identify, in part because the person using the drugs may be hiding a drug problem. If you suspect someone has overdosed, or if you suspect someone is experiencing withdrawal, give first aid as described below.

If someone has accidentally swallowed an overdose of medication, or if a medication was taken by the wrong person, see **Poison** on page 163.

A Guide to Drugs

All drugs fall within certain broad categories, based upon their origin and the effects they have on the body. Depending upon what form they are in, drugs can be eaten, smoked, injected, or inhaled.

Illegal drugs vary greatly in purity and quality, so the buyer never knows if the drug is what it is represented to be. Many drug overdoses result when drugs are diluted, or "cut," with another chemical. A drug user accustomed to diluted drugs may also unknowingly use a purer, more potent drug.

Marijuana, *hash*, and *hash oil* are all made from the plant *Cannabis sativa*. These drugs give the user a sense of euphoria and distort his or her perception of time and space. They also impair coordination and concentration and can slow the user's responses even after the initial high has worn off. Excessive use can cause memory loss and fatigue.

Stimulants ("uppers") are drugs that stimulate the central nervous system. They relieve fatigue and give the user a feeling of well-being. They also increase heart and breathing rates and raise the user's blood pressure. High doses can cause hyperactivity, combative behavior, stroke, collapse, and death. Long-term users can develop psychotic symptoms (loss of touch with reality) and health problems; frequent use of large amounts can cause brain damage. *Amphetamines* are stimulants. "Ice" is a smokeable form of amphetamine; seizures and paranoia are common side effects.

Depressants ("downers") are drugs that slow down the body's functions. In small amounts they promote calmness and relax muscles; in larger quantities they can cause confusion, delusions, loss of coordination, collapse, coma, and death. *Barbiturates*, *sedatives*, *hypnotics*, and *tranquilizers* are all depressants.

Alcohol is not a medication but it is a depressant. A small amount of alcohol relieves inhibitions; larger amounts can cause rowdy behavior, slurred speech, double vision, vomiting, poor judgment, loss of coordination, and slowed reflexes; very large amounts can cause blackouts and seizures and can stop breathing. Alcohol damages the central nervous system; long-term use damages the liver and brain.

Narcotics are drugs that are used for their anesthetic effects. They are available in a wide variety of forms and can be extremely addictive. *Opium* is a narcotic, as are all of its derivatives: *morphine*,

Signs and Symptoms

Overdose

- Agitation; violent behavior; terror
- Hallucinations
- Sweating
- Drowsiness
- Difficulty breathing
- Nausea; vomiting
- Abnormal pupil size (either very large or very small)
- Seizures
- Unconsciousness

codeine, and *heroin*. Heroin gives the user a "rush" when taken; it also can cause breathing problems, coma, and death.

Cocaine is derived from the coca plant and is available in many forms, including *freebase* and *crack*. Cocaine alters the user's mental state and produces a temporary sense of euphoria followed by a deep depression. The higher the high, the lower the low that follows. Cocaine can also cause anxiety, hallucinations, paranoia, spasms, seizures, heart attack, stroke, breathing emergencies, and death. Long-term users may experience cocaine psychosis.

Hallucinogens, also called *psychedelics*, are mind-altering drugs that distort the user's perceptions — he or she may "see" sounds and "hear" colors. Their effects are unpredictable. Hallucinogens can intensify psychological problems and cause "bad trips." After the immediate effects of the drug wear off, the user may still have "flashbacks" and show signs of psychosis. The physical effects of hallucinogens include high blood pressure, dilated pupils, tremors, wild behavior, muscle weakness, and elevated body temperature. *LSD*, *mescaline* (from the peyote plant), and *psilocybin* are all hallucinogens. *PCP* ("angel dust") was developed as an anesthetic but can cause hallucinations, violent and bizarre behavior, psychosis, and death.

Inhalants are breathable chemicals that have mind-altering or aphrodisiac effects. Inhalants provide a brief "rush." To sustain a high, the user must inhale the chemical repeatedly, which intensifies the danger. Inhalants can cause incoherence, staggering, violent behavior, suffocation, collapse, and heart failure. Long-term use can cause permanent damage to internal organs and the central nervous system. Most of the substances that are abused are not intended to be used as inhalants — for example, glue, gasoline, cleaning fluid, spray products, and nail polish remover. Some inhalants are legitimate drugs — for example, *nitrous oxide* ("laughing gas") and *amyl nitrate* (prescribed for angina)—that are abused. *Butyl nitrate* is a nonprescription inhalant sold in shops that sell drug paraphernalia.

"Actalikes" are street drugs that act like certain legitimate counterparts. "Lookalikes" are street drugs that look like certain legal counterparts. Both often contain poisonous substances. Since these drugs are manufactured illegally, the user cannot know exactly what he or she is taking.

Withdrawal

- Depression
- Extreme restlessness
- Tremors
- Anxiety; agitation
- Nausea; vomiting
- Cold sweat
- Hallucinations; delusions
- Seizures

FIRST AID

Overdose or Withdrawal

- Call EMS.
- If you suspect withdrawal, try to find out what drug the victim has been taking.
- If you suspect overdose, try to find out what drug was taken, when it was taken, how it was taken (by mouth, injection, etc.), and how much. Be aware that the user may have taken more than one drug. Collect samples of the drug or of the user's vomit for analysis.
- Call your local Poison Control Center for advice.

DO NOT try to reason with someone who is on drugs. Do not expect him or her to behave reasonably.

DO NOT try to keep the user awake.

DO NOT offer your opinions when offering assistance. You don't need to know why drugs were taken to give first aid.

DO NOT jeopardize your own safety. Some drugs can cause violent and unpredictable behavior. Get professional help.

1. Check the victim's ABCs. Open the airway; check breathing and circulation.

    If the ABCs are not present, begin CPR at once. (See the Emergency Action Guides on pages 199–210.)

    If the victim is unconscious but breathing, place him or her in the recovery position. (See page 183.)

    If the victim is conscious, loosen the victim's clothing, keep him or her warm, and provide reassurance. Try to keep the victim calm. If you suspect an overdose, try to prevent the victim from taking more drugs.

2. If the victim develops signs of shock (including pale, clammy skin, weakness, bluish lips and fingernails, and decreasing alertness), give first aid for shock. (See **Shock** on page 172.)

3. If the victim starts having seizures, protect him or her from injury and give first aid for convulsions. (See **Seizures** on page 168.)

4. Continue to monitor the victim's ABCs until you have medical help. Don't leave him or her alone.

More on the Subject

Someone who has become dependent on a drug probably won't be able to stop without experiencing withdrawal symptoms. Withdrawal is best accomplished with professional help. Drug rehabilitation may require emotional and medical help in a drug-free environment.

Ear Injury

The *outer ear* collects sound waves and directs them through the *ear canal* to the *middle ear*. From there they go into the *inner ear*, where they are translated into nerve impulses and transmitted to the brain. The inner ear also controls our sense of balance. Both hearing and balance can be disrupted by an injury or illness that affects the ear.

The *eardrum* separates the outer ear from the middle ear, and the *eustachian tube* runs from the inner ear to the throat. These parts of the ear are sensitive to pressure (Figure 66).

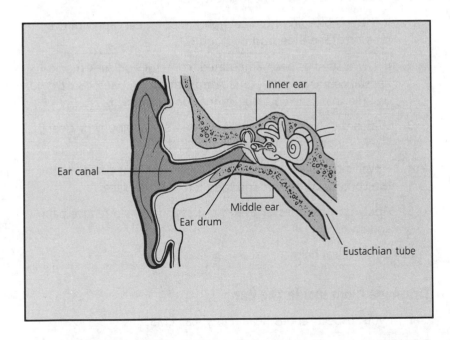

Figure 66
The anatomy of the ear

Any problem with your middle or inner ear means that you need medical attention. Special instruments are needed to examine the ear completely. More important, a lack of treatment can lead to loss of hearing. The workings of the inner ear are intimately connected to the brain. That's one reason it's important to apply a sterile dressing over an injured ear until you get medical help.

In general, ears should be treated with great care. Never put *anything* in the ear canal without first consulting a physician, and never thump the head to try to correct an ear problem.

If the ear is frostbitten, see **Cold Exposure** on page 117.

Signs and Symptoms

- Swelling; redness; bruising; bleeding from the visible part of the ear
- Pain; earache
- Impaired hearing
- Dizziness; vertigo; loss of balance
- Nausea; vomiting

FIRST AID

Injury to the Outer Ear

- If you suspect serious head injury, call EMS.

1. If there is bleeding from cuts on the outer ear, apply direct pressure. (See **Bleeding** on page 62.)

2. If any tissue has been amputated, collect it and seek medical assistance immediately. (See **Amputation** on page 48.) *Do not* assume that severed tissue cannot be reattached.

3. Watch the injured ear for drainage — either bloody or clear fluid — from the ear canal (see below).

4. Cover the entire ear with a sterile dressing that conforms to the contour of the ear and tape it loosely in place.

5. Apply cold compresses over the dressing to help reduce pain and swelling.

6. Get medical help.

FIRST AID

Drainage from Inside the Ear

- If you suspect serious head injury, call EMS.

DO NOT block any drainage coming from the ear.
DO NOT try to clean drainage inside the ear.

1. Cover the outside of the ear with a sterile dressing that conforms to the contour of the ear and tape it loosely in place.

2. To promote drainage, have the victim lie down on his or her side with the affected ear down. *Do not* move the victim if you suspect any neck or back injury.

3. Get medical help.

Foreign Body Stuck in the Ear

DO NOT try to remove a foreign body from the ear unless you can see it clearly.

1. Calm and reassure the victim, who may be very disturbed.

2. Look inside the ear.
   If you can clearly see the foreign body at the entrance to the ear canal and the victim is cooperative, turn the victim's head so the affected ear points down and gently remove the object with tweezers. Then get medical help to be sure the entire object was removed.
   If you think a small object may be lodged within the ear, but you cannot see it, do not reach inside the ear canal with tweezers. You might push the object further in or may cause hearing damage. Get medical help.
   If an insect is in the ear, don't let the victim poke a finger in his or her ear, since this may make the insect bite or sting.
   First turn the victim's head so that the affected ear is up and wait to see if the insect crawls out.
   If this doesn't work, if medical help is not nearby, and if the victim is in intense pain, place a few drops of room-temperature oil (mineral oil, baby oil, cooking oil, or olive oil) in the ear canal to drown the insect. Then get medical help. Use oil only if you are certain that the foreign body is an insect, since oil can cause other kinds of objects to swell.

Ruptured Eardrum

The eardrum can be ruptured by a blow to the head, an object poked into the ear, a blast of noise or an explosion, an ear infection, or a deep dive. If the eardrum has been ruptured, dirt and bacteria from the outer ear canal can pass through the ruptured eardrum into the inner ear.

If you suspect the victim may have a ruptured eardrum (there is severe pain), place sterile cotton gently in the outer ear canal to keep the inside of the ear clean and get medical help.

Electrical Injury

Any direct contact with electrical current — household current, high-voltage current, or lightning — is potentially fatal. The human body is a good conductor of electricity, and electrical current can go right through it, injuring both the skin and internal organs. Electrical burns may look minor, but there may be serious internal problems. If electrical current passes through the heart, it can cause heart damage; if it passes through the brain stem, it can knock the victim unconscious or cause the victim to stop breathing.

Electrical current takes the path of least resistance. Wood and rubber do not conduct electricity well; water and metal do. Household current usually causes only skin burns, but if the victim is in contact with water when he or she is electrocuted (for example, standing on damp ground, sitting in the bathtub, or handling an electrical appliance with wet hands), the effects are much more severe. Injuries from contact with electrical current of over 110 volts should be assumed to be serious until proven otherwise.

The severity of electrical injuries depends upon the strength of the current, how long the victim was exposed to it, how much protection or insulation he or she had, and the path the current took through the victim's body. Alternating current (AC) is more injurious than direct current (DC) because it causes the muscles to go into prolonged spasms.

Signs and Symptoms

- Unpleasant tingling or sense of having been shaken; severe jolt
- Skin burns where electricity entered and exited the body. (These burns may be painless, since nerves are damaged.)
- Mouth burns (from putting a "live" extension cord in the mouth)
- Muscular pain; fatigue; headache
- Momentary or prolonged loss of consciousness
- Respiratory failure
- Cardiopulmonary arrest

Electrocution

FIRST AID

- Shut off the electrical current. (See box on page 134).
- Call EMS.

DO NOT touch the skin of someone who is being electrocuted.
DO NOT get within 20 feet of someone who is being electrocuted by high-voltage electrical current until the power is turned off.
DO NOT move a victim of electrical injury unless there is immediate danger.

1. Check the victim's ABCs. Open the airway; check breathing and circulation. If necessary, begin rescue breathing, CPR, or bleeding control. (See the Emergency Action Guides on pages 199–210.)

   If the ABCs are present but the victim is unconscious, give first aid for unconsciousness. (See **Unconsciousness** on page 182.)

2. Locate the entry and exit burns, if possible, and check the victim for any other injuries. Give first aid for the most serious injuries first.

3. Take steps to prevent shock. Lay the victim flat, elevate the feet 8 to 12 inches, and cover the victim with a coat or blanket. *Do not* place the victim in the shock position if you suspect any head, neck, back, or leg injury or if the position causes the victim discomfort. (See **Shock** on page 172.)

4. Give first aid for the entry and exit burns. Treat all electrical burns as severe burns. (See **Burns** on page 84.)

5. Stay with the victim until EMS arrives.

How to Rescue Someone Who Is Being Electrocuted

Someone who is in direct contact with electrical current needs help *immediately*. The victim may be unconscious, or he or she may be unable to move because of muscle spasms.

Rescuing a victim of electrical injury is dangerous. If you touch the skin of the victim, you too could be electrocuted. Do not become a second victim!

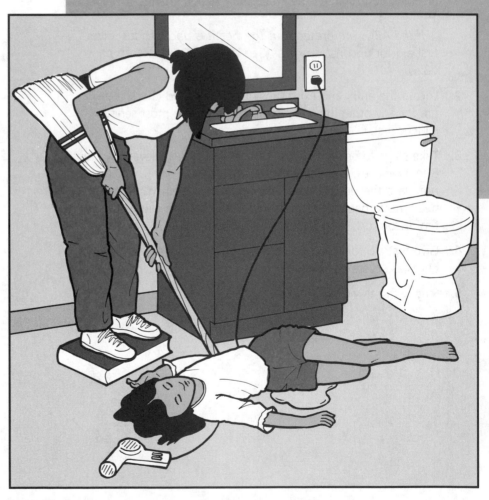

Figure 67
Standing on dry material to separate a victim from current

Accidents Involving Household Current

To stop the flow of current to the victim, first make sure you are not near or in water. Then unplug the appliance (just turning it off, even by a wall switch, is not sufficient) or turn off the main power switch (do not waste time trying to find the exact fuse or circuit breaker).

If you cannot turn off the current, you may try to push the victim away from the current (or the current away from the victim) if it is safe to do so. Making sure you are not near electrified water, stand on some kind of dry insulating material (a rubber door mat, a pile of newspapers, a thick book) and use a dry wooden object (pole, board, chair) to separate the victim from the current (Figure 67). *Do not* use an object that will conduct electricity to you (including anything damp or made of metal). An alternative is to loop a dry rope (or dry fabric or pantyhose) around the victim's arm or leg and use it to pull the victim free of the current.

Accidents Involving High-Voltage Current

If someone is being electrocuted by high-voltage current, do not go near him or her. High voltage currents can arc (jump) as far as 20 feet, and normal types of insulation will not protect you. Place an emergency call to the power company to have the power turned off.

If someone is inside a car near a downed power line, tell him or her to stay inside the car until the power is turned off. If the individual leaves the car, he or she risks being electrocuted.

The eye is delicate and extremely complicated (Figure 68). All eye problems are serious because they can lead to loss of sight or infection. As a lay rescuer, your priority is to do no further harm and to take whatever steps possible to protect the victim's sight.

Nontraumatic eye problems—for example, disease or infection—do not require first aid but do require medical attention. The eye also can be harmed by certain prescription medications as well as medical conditions (for example, diabetes and hypertension). Eye problems can be an indication of head injury or problems with the brain.

It's important to get prompt medical attention for all eye problems; the eye is easily damaged, and special instruments are needed to examine the eye completely. A delay in getting medical attention can cause irreversible loss of sight.

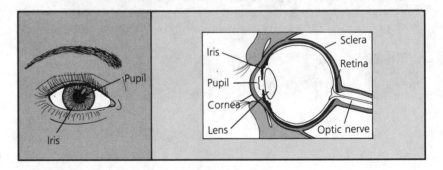

Figure 68
Anatomy of the eye

Signs and Symptoms

- Cuts, bruises, or other signs of direct trauma
- Stinging and burning; pain in or around the eye
- Redness; bloodshot appearance
- Dryness; scratchiness; itchiness
- Foreign body visible in the eye; sensation of something being in the eye
- Discharge; tears; rapid blinking
- Sensitivity to light
- Double vision; impaired vision; loss of sight (with or without pain or signs of injury)
- Headache
- Pupils of unequal size

How to Flush the Eye with Water

The safest way to deal with a foreign body or substance in the eye is to flush the eye liberally with sterile saline solution. If you have no saline solution, use tap water. If the victim is wearing contact lenses, don't remove them before flushing the eye.

1. Tilt the victim's head so that the affected eye is down. Be careful not to touch or contaminate the unaffected eye.
2. With one hand, pour a steady stream of water from the inside corner of the eye (next to the nose) to the outside corner (Figure 69).
3. With your other hand, hold the victim's eyelid open to make sure the eye is properly flushed. Keep flushing the eye for 15 to 30 minutes, or until you have medical help.

   If both eyes are affected, have the victim open his or her eyes underwater in a bowl of fresh water. If you are washing chemicals from the victim's eyes, use a stream of fresh water. (If possible, put the victim in a shower.)
   Remove contact lenses after flushing.

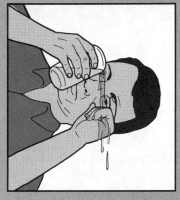

Figure 69
Flushing the eye

Foreign Body in the Eye

A foreign body in the eye may not be visible. Sometimes a scratch on the surface of the eye gives the sensation of something in the eye, when in fact nothing is there.

- If the eye injury is serious, call EMS.

DO NOT press on an injured eye or allow the victim to rub his or her eye.

DO NOT remove contact lenses unless rapid swelling is occurring or you cannot get prompt medical help.

DO NOT attempt to remove a foreign body that is resting on the iris or pupil or that appears to be embedded in any part of the eye. Get medical help.

DO NOT use dry cotton (including cotton swabs) or sharp instruments (including tweezers) on the eye.

FIRST AID

1. Wash your hands thoroughly.
2. Examine the affected eye in good light. To help locate the foreign body, have the victim look all around as you examine the eye.
3. If you can't find the foreign body, look inside the victim's lower eyelid. Have the victim look up as you gently pull down his or her lower lid. If you can see the object on the inner surface of the eyelid, try to flush it out with water (see box on page 137) or to lift it off with a clean cloth (not a tissue or cotton swab). If you are unable to remove the object using these methods, get medical help.
4. If you are still unable to find the object, examine the inside of the upper lid (see box opposite). If the foreign body can be seen on the inner surface of the upper eyelid, try to flush it out with water (see box on page 137) or to lift it off with a clean cloth (not a tissue or cotton swab). If you cannot remove the object using these methods, get medical help.
5. If you cannot locate the foreign body, or if you remove it but the victim still has discomfort (pain, tears, blurred vision), cover *both* eyes with eye patches or dry, protective dressings (this will discourage eye movement) and get medical help. Having the eyes bandaged can be frightening, so remember to calm and reassure the victim.

More on the Subject

If after having something removed from the eye, the victim develops any of the signs and symptoms on page 136, get medical help.

FIRST AID

Object Stuck in the Eye

Any penetrating injury of the eye requires immediate medical attention, even if the object in the eye is small.

- If the eye injury is serious, call EMS.

DO NOT attempt to remove the embedded object.
DO NOT press on the injured eye or allow the victim to rub his or her eye.
DO NOT remove contact lenses unless rapid swelling is occurring or you cannot get prompt medical help.

1. Leave the stuck object in place. *Do not* touch it and *do not* let anything press on it.

How to Inspect the Inside of the Upper Eyelid

If a foreign body is inside the upper eyelid, here is how to get a closer look.

1. Have the victim look down (and keep looking down during this entire procedure).
2. Lay a clean, smooth stick such as a cotton swab or coffee stirrer horizontally across the victim's upper eyelid (Figure 70a).
3. Gently grasp the upper eyelashes.
4. Fold the eyelid back over the swab by pulling on the eyelashes (Figure 70b).

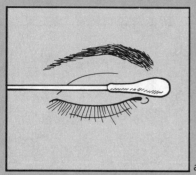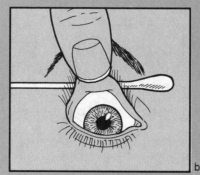

Figure 70 a, b
Inspecting the inside of the upper eyelid

5. After you have removed the foreign body by flushing the eye or by using a clean cloth, flip the eyelid back again.

2. Wash your hands thoroughly.

3. How you bandage the eye depends upon the size of the object embedded in it.

    If the object is large, place a paper cup or cone over the injured eye and tape it in place. Cover the uninjured eye with an eye patch or a sterile dressing.

    If the object is small, cover both eyes with eye patches or sterile dressings.

4. Calm and reassure the victim. Having both eyes bandaged can be frightening.

5. Keep the victim quiet until you have medical help.

How to Remove Contact Lenses

You can remove both hard and soft contact lenses using the following steps:

1. Wash your hands thoroughly.
2. With one thumb, hold the victim's upper eyelid open.
3. Have the victim look toward his or her nose with the affected eye.
4. Use your other thumb to slide the contact toward the white area at the outside corner of the eye (Figure 71a).
5. Pull the skin at the outside corner of the eye down and out (Figure 71b). The lens should pop free.

   If you have any difficulty removing a lens, get medical help.

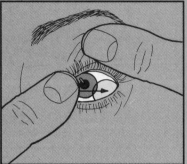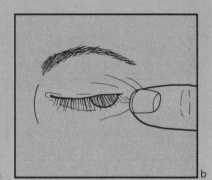

Figure 71 a, b
Removing a contact lens

FIRST AID

Chemical Exposure

If harmful chemicals—dry or wet—get into the eye, give first aid *immediately*. The eyes are more sensitive to chemicals than the skin. Even if you are not sure that the chemical is harmful, flush the eye(s) thoroughly and get medical help.

- If the eye injury is serious, call EMS.
- Try to determine the type of chemical. Then call your local Poison Control Center for advice.

DO NOT press an injured eye or let the victim rub his or her eye(s).

1. Flush the eye with lots of fresh water (see box on page 137) for at least 15 to 30 minutes, or until you have medical help. You may have to force the victim's eyes open.

2. If both eyes are affected, or if other parts of the victim's body are affected, have the victim take a shower.

3. Take out contact lenses (see box opposite) after the eyes have been thoroughly rinsed.

4. Cover both eyes with eye patches or sterile dressings until you have medical help. Even if only one eye is affected, covering both eyes will help discourage eye movement.

Burns

A blast of hot air or steam can burn the face and eyes. Natural sun and tanning lamps can cause burns to the cornea. The seriousness of an eye burn may not be apparent for 24 hours.

- If the eye injury is serious, call EMS.

DO NOT press an injured eye or let the victim rub his or her eye. DO NOT let the burn become contaminated. Avoid breathing or coughing on the burned area.

1. Immediately flush the eyes with cool water to reduce swelling and relieve pain. If flushing makes the pain worse, *stop*.

2. A light, cool compress may be helpful, but *do not* apply pressure and *do not* use a fluffy (cotton) bandage.

3. If the white of the eye or the area around the eye swells, or if the victim experiences any visual problems, get medical help.

Cuts and Blows to the Eye

Direct trauma to the eye can injure the area around the eye, the surface of the eyeball, or the inner eye.

- If the eye injury is serious, call EMS.

DO NOT press on an injured eye or allow the victim to rub his or her eye.

1. If the eyeball is, or may have been, injured, get medical help immediately. Suspect that the surface of the eye may have been scratched if the victim was wearing contact lenses when the trauma occurred or if there is a cut on the eyelid.

2. If a "black eye" is forming, gently apply cold compresses immediately to reduce swelling and help stop the bleeding. *Do not* use raw steak.

3. If there are cuts about the eye, apply sterile dressings. *Do not* use fluffy (cotton) dressings, and *do not* apply pressure to control bleeding.

4. Sometimes bleeding into the inside of the eye will cause a pool of blood to form behind the cornea. A layer of blood will be visible inside the iris (Figure 72) when the victim's head is raised. If this occurs, cover both of the victim's eyes with sterile dressings, keep him or her quiet, and get medical help immediately.

Figure 72
Bleeding inside the eye

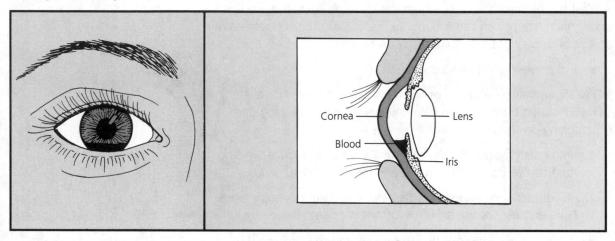

Facial Injury

Facial injuries include cuts, broken facial bones, and broken teeth. Trauma to the mouth may cause bleeding or swelling, which can lead to obstruction of the airway and difficulty breathing.

If the victim has injured his or her ear(s), see **Ear Injury** on page 129.
If the victim has injured his or her eye(s), see **Eye Injury** on page 136.
If the victim has injured his or her nose, see **Nose Injury** on page 160.

Signs and Symptoms

- Obvious cuts, bruises, scrapes, bleeding, or swelling
- Misshapen appearance of face

- Injured jaw. (Signs and symptoms include facial pain, ear pain, swelling, difficulty speaking or opening and closing the mouth, and difficulty swallowing.)
- Loose, broken, or missing teeth; broken dentures or dental work
- Sensation of a swollen airway; obstructed airway
- Bleeding from the mouth or bleeding into the throat

Facial Injury

- If the victim is seriously injured, call EMS.
- Remember to keep the victim's airway clear — it may become obstructed by saliva, blood, vomit, swollen or lacerated tissues, broken teeth, dirt, broken dental work or dentures, or foreign objects.

DO NOT overlook the possibility of serious head injury and neck injury, even if the victim's facial injuries seem minor.

DO NOT give the victim anything by mouth.

DO NOT move misshapen facial bones.

DO NOT throw away a tooth that has been knocked out. Save it for possible reimplantation. (Baby teeth may not be reimplanted.)

1. Check the victim's ABCs. Open the airway; check breathing and circulation. If necessary, begin rescue breathing, CPR, or bleeding control. (See the Emergency Action Guides on pages 199–210.) Mouth injuries and jaw fractures can make it difficult to give rescue breathing; instead of using mouth-to-mouth resuscitation, you may need to use mouth-to-nose breathing.

   If the ABCs are present but the victim is unconscious, give first aid for head injury. (See **Head Injury** on page 147.)

2. Try to determine whether or not spinal injury may have occurred. Signs and symptoms of spinal injury include back or neck pain; numbness, tingling, or loss of sensation in the arms or legs; and inability to move parts of the body at will. (See **Spinal Injury** on page 175.) If you are in doubt, or if the victim is unconscious, assume spinal injury has occurred.

   If spinal injury is not suspected, place the victim in the recovery position (see page 183) to allow fluids to drain. If the victim is conscious, an alternative is to have him or her sit down and lean forward.

3. Clear the victim's airway of any fluids or debris with a finger sweep. If there is severe bleeding in the mouth and you have a suction bulb, suction out the blood. If the airway is still obstructed, give first aid for choking. (See the Emergency Action Guides on pages 199–210.) Continue to monitor the victim's airway and to keep it clear.

4. Monitor the victim for signs of serious head injury. Signs and symptoms include severe headache, severe or persistent vomiting, confusion or lapses in alertness, vision problems, and convulsions. (See **Head Injury** on page 147.) If the victim has severe facial injuries and is not talking, or claims not to be in much pain, suspect that judgment has been impaired by serious head injury.

5. Control severe facial or mouth bleeding by applying direct pressure. (See **Bleeding** on page 62.) If you suspect broken facial bones, apply pressure gently.

6. Administer first aid for wounds as needed. (See **Wounds** on page 186.)

7. If the victim may have broken his or her jaw, do not put anything in his or her mouth. Apply cold compresses to help relieve the pain and stop the bleeding. If possible, have the victim hold the jaw in place until you have medical help. If the victim vomits, support the jaw.

8. Care for any dental injuries (see box).

9. Seek medical and dental care as needed.

More on the Subject

Wounds to the face can be disfiguring and often are treated differently from wounds elsewhere. Special attention is given to the cause of the wound and the plane of the face.

Check to see if the victim's tetanus immunization is current.

How to Care for Dental Injuries

Here are the general first aid measures for dental injuries in a conscious victim:

1. Save any teeth that have been knocked out for possible reimplantation.
2. Apply cold compresses for pain.
3. Apply direct pressure to control bleeding.
4. Seek dental attention immediately.

If a baby tooth has been knocked out, it may not be reimplanted. However, you should save it and call your dentist immediately. Pick up the tooth by the chewing edge. Do not touch or rub the root. Place it in a container of cool milk or water and cover. Apply cold compresses to the injured area to help relieve the pain and stop the bleeding. Give the child nothing by mouth for 2 hours to give a clot time to form. If pain or bleeding persist, call the dentist.

If an adult tooth has been knocked out, reimplantation may be possible. Pick up the tooth by the chewing edge. Do not touch or rub the root. Place the tooth back in the tooth socket, and press it into place. If this is not possible, rinse the tooth with water and, if possible, put it in a container of cool milk or water and cover, or wrap it in a sterile gauze pad or clean cloth that has been soaked in milk. If this also is not possible, lay the tooth inside the victim's cheek. It's important to keep the tooth with the victim. The sooner dental attention is received, the better chances are for successful reimplantation.

To control bleeding, place a sterile gauze pad in the injured tooth socket and have the victim apply pressure by biting down. You may also apply cool used teabags; the tannic acid in the tea helps stop the bleeding.

If a tooth is cracked, cover it with a sterile gauze pad and compress it firmly. Crunchy, sweet, or hot foods or liquids should be avoided until the tooth is fixed.

If dental work is broken, do not pull it out. If it falls out by itself, remove it from the victim's mouth and save it.

If dentures are broken and loose, remove them or have the victim spit them out. Broken pieces of denture could fall back into the throat and obstruct the airway. If the broken dentures have not been loosened, leave them alone.

Fainting   *See Unconsciousness*

Fever   *See Seizures*

Foot Injury   *See Bone, Joint, and Muscle Injuries*

Fracture   *See Bone, Joint, and Muscle Injuries*

Frostbite   *See Cold Exposure*

Genital Injury

The genital area in both men and women has many nerves and blood vessels, which means that genital injuries can be very painful and can bleed heavily. The genital area is structurally complicated, and genital injuries can affect the reproductive organs as well as the bladder and urethra.

Any pain or swelling in the genital area requires immediate medical attention. In little girls, discomfort can be caused by a foreign body lodged in the vagina.

Be aware that genital injuries are sometimes the result of assault, rape, or sexual abuse. You do not need to know exactly what happened in order to give first aid, but if you suspect rape or sexual abuse, try not to disturb possible evidence, and seek medical assistance immediately.

If the victim has a zipper injury, see **Wounds** on page 186.

Signs and Symptoms

- Extreme pain
- Swelling
- Bruises
- Bleeding
- Change in shape
- Object embedded in a body opening or wound
- Urine leakage

FIRST AID

Genital Injury

- If the victim is seriously injured, or if you think an assault or abuse has occurred, call EMS.

DO NOT allow the victim to walk unless absolutely necessary.

DO NOT overlook the possibility of internal bleeding.

DO NOT volunteer your opinions about the circumstances.

DO NOT accuse or confront the victim.

DO NOT disturb possible evidence of assault or abuse unless a medical emergency exists. If you suspect assault or abuse, do not allow the victim to change clothes, bathe, or shower.

1. Calm and reassure the victim. As you give first aid, maintain privacy for the victim and shield the injured area.

2. Use direct pressure to control external bleeding. (See **Bleeding** on page 62.) Place a sterile dressing over any open wounds. (See **Wounds** on page 186.) If there is severe bleeding from the vagina, pack the area with sterile gauze or clean washcloths.

3. Apply cold compresses to reduce swelling.

4. If the testicles have been injured, support them with a sling made from folded towels laid across the victim's thighs.

5. If an object is embedded in a body opening or wound, leave it alone. Removing it may cause further damage.

6. Get medical help.

More on the Subject

In cases of rape or sexual abuse, a medical examination is essential, in part because it can prevent the spread of certain diseases.

Hand Injury *See Bone, Joint, and Muscle Injuries*

Head Injury

A serious head injury can involve one or all the elements of your head: the scalp, skull, brain, spinal fluid, and blood vessels (Figure 73). Head injury can be external, internal, or both. Even if your skull is not fractured, your brain can bang against the inside of the skull and be damaged. If there is bleeding within the skull, complications may follow.

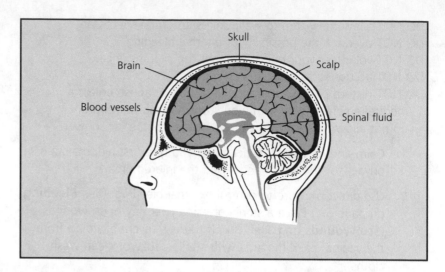

Figure 73
Anatomy of the head

Head injury is often associated with neck injury, since a blow that is forceful enough to injure the head is also likely to affect the neck. Always suspect neck injury when there has been trauma to the head. (See **Spinal Injury** on page 175.)

If a child is up and running immediately after getting a bump on the head, serious head injury is highly unlikely. However, the child should still be closely watched for the next 24 hours, since sometimes signs and symptoms of head injury can be delayed.

If the victim has an injured ear, see **Ear Injury** on page 129.
If the victim has an injured eye, see **Eye Injury** on page 136.
If the victim has an injured face, see **Facial Injury** on page 142.
If the victim has an injured nose, see **Nose Injury** on page 160.

Signs and Symptoms

- Obvious signs of trauma, such as a dent or fracture in the skull, a wound in the scalp, and bleeding. (The amount of bleeding may not tell you much about the size or severity of the wound.)
- Severe headache that is not relieved by over-the-counter headache remedies
- Severe or persistent vomiting
- Dazed or confused behavior; lapses in alertness or consciousness, either immediately following the accident or developing later
- Personality changes, such as increased restlessness or irritability
- Increased drowsiness (for example, if the victim is sleepy at a time he or she normally would not be)

- Slurred speech
- Stiff neck
- Convulsions
- Difficulty seeing; double vision; pupils of unequal size
- Weakness in an arm or leg
- Fluid draining from the ears, nose, or mouth; bleeding from the nose or mouth that isn't the result of a facial injury
- Slowing of the rate of breathing
- In infants: swelling of the fontanel ("soft spot" on the skull at the top of the head)

Head Injury

- If you suspect serious head injury, call EMS.
- Suspect neck injury. Unless it is absolutely critical, don't move the victim; keep him or her in the position found. If the victim is in urgent danger and you must move him or her *immediately*, see How to Move a Victim with a Suspected Spinal Injury on page 178.
- Try to find out what happened. If you cannot rely on the victim to tell you, look for clues and ask bystanders.

DO NOT let other, more obvious, injuries distract you from the head injury.

DO NOT move the victim unless absolutely necessary.

DO NOT shake the victim because he or she seems dazed.

DO NOT pick up a fallen child with any sign of head injury.

DO NOT remove any object sticking in a wound.

1. Check the victim's ABCs. Open the airway; check breathing and circulation. If necessary, begin rescue breathing, CPR, or bleeding control. (See the Emergency Action Guides on pages 199–210.)

    If the ABCs are present but the victim is unconscious, care for the victim as if there is a spinal injury. Stabilize the head and neck by placing your hands on both sides of the victim's head, keeping the head in line with the spine and preventing movement. Wait for medical help.

    If the victim is conscious, keep him or her calm. Encourage the victim to lie still and not to attempt to get up. Protect the victim's neck from activity, motion, and harmful objects. Be aware that blows to the head can leave a victim disoriented, confused, or combative.

If the victim cannot remember all that happened, he or she probably was briefly unconscious. Inform EMS personnel or the physician when the victim is examined.

2. Give first aid for any obvious head injuries.

   If you suspect the skull may be fractured, do not apply direct pressure to the bleeding site and do not remove any debris from the wound. Cover the wound with sterile gauze dressings and get medical help immediately.

   For superficial scalp wounds, use a clean bandage, cloth, or towel and apply direct pressure. Continuous pressure will almost always stop bleeding. (See **Bleeding** on page 62.) Give first aid for wounds as needed. (See **Wounds** on page 186.)

3. If the victim starts having seizures, protect the head by placing cushions around it. Remove any harmful objects from the area and give first aid for convulsions. (See **Seizures** on page 168.)

4. Vomiting is common with head injuries. Take steps to protect the victim's airway. (See box opposite.) Children often vomit once after a head injury. But even if the child does not vomit again and is not behaving differently, contact your physician.

5. Apply ice to areas of swelling.

6. Get medical help if the victim shows any of the signs and symptoms on page 151. It is always a good idea to have the victim of a head injury examined by a physician, even if the injury appears minor.

More on the Subject

It is important to observe the victim for at least 24 hours following head trauma. Sometimes there is no evidence of serious head injury early on, but signs and symptoms develop later. It is best if someone who knows the victim stays with him or her to watch for changes in behavior, which may be subtle.

Someone with head trauma may have a mild headache, nausea, and want to sleep. Do not try to prevent the victim from going to sleep. However, do awaken the victim every 2 to 3 hours and check for alertness. Ask the victim specific questions, such as an address, the name of the family dog, etc.

When observing someone for the signs and symptoms of head injury, do not complicate the situation by allowing him or her to consume alcohol within 48 hours of the accident. Offer the victim foods

Vomiting

Vomiting is not a medical emergency, but it can happen along with many emergency conditions. Vomiting occurs when the stomach muscles suddenly contract and "throw up" the stomach contents.

Sometimes, a victim inhales vomit. That can lead to choking or lung complications. To minimize this risk, do the following:

- When a conscious victim throws up, lean the victim forward and support his or her forehead.
- Be aware that unconscious victims often throw up. If you do not suspect spinal injury, place an unconscious victim in the recovery position (see page 183); if the victim vomits, this will allow fluids to drain.
- When a victim with suspected neck injury vomits, support his or her head and neck and roll the victim to one side. This is best accomplished with the help of several bystanders. (See page 177.)

Vomiting can be a sign of serious injury or illness. Get medical help immediately if:

- The vomit contains bright-red blood, yellow or green material, or dark material that looks like coffee grounds.
- Vomiting follows an injury to the abdomen, or is accompanied by severe abdominal pain, or the abdomen is tender to the touch.
- The victim vomits more than once after a recent head trauma.
- Vomiting is persistent or is associated with diarrhea, especially in an infant.
- The victim vomits and has signs of dehydration, including dry mouth, sunken eyes, severe thirst, a decrease in the usual amount of urine, and irritability.
- A child recovering from the flu or chicken pox has persistent vomiting along with behavioral changes.

that are easy to digest. Since medication can affect alertness, the victim should take only prescribed medications during this period. Have him or her refrain from vigorous activity for 24 hours.

If the victim becomes unusually drowsy, develops a severe headache or stiff neck, vomits more than once, becomes confused, or behaves abnormally, get medical help immediately.

The heart is a muscle that acts as a pump. With each contraction (heartbeat), your heart sends blood in 2 directions: oxygen-poor blood goes to the lungs, and oxygen-rich blood goes to all parts of the body. To work effectively, your heart needs to have enough oxygenated blood within its own tissue, an adequate supply of blood to pump to the rest of the body, and proper electrical stimulation to cause it to beat.

Sometimes the heart does not get enough oxygen to support its workload. (This can happen for many reasons, including narrow or blocked coronary arteries, low blood pressure, or too little oxygen in the blood.) This can lead to an attack of *angina pectoris* (temporary chest pain) or a true *heart attack*. An angina attack may be relieved by lessening the demands on the heart, usually through rest and medication. If an angina attack is not relieved, it can lead to a heart attack.

During a heart attack (technically known as a *myocardial infarction*, or MI), the muscle of the heart itself is damaged. This in turn can lead to *heart failure* (in which the heart does not function effectively), *fibrillating* (in which the heart quivers instead of pumping strongly), or *cardiac arrest* (in which the heart stops beating altogether). These conditions can be fatal — but much can be done to alleviate them if the victim receives expert medical attention quickly. EMS personnel can rapidly administer oxygen and medication that increases the blood flow to the heart; new treatments include clot-thinning medications and electrical defibrillation.

Medical attention is essential for anyone who shows any of the signs or symptoms of a heart attack, even a person who dismisses the problem or doesn't seem a likely candidate for a heart attack. Although chest pain can be caused by many different conditions, anyone experiencing it needs expert medical attention to rule out the possibility of heart disease.

Heart attacks and strokes are sometimes mistaken for each other. (See **Stroke** on page 181.) A stroke is a circulation problem within the brain. A heart attack can cause a stroke.

Signs and Symptoms

Most heart attack victims have one or more of the following symptoms:

- Discomfort or pressure in the center of the chest, ranging from an ache to a crushing sensation ("like someone sitting on my chest"). The pain sometimes extends to the jaw(s), shoulder(s), or arm(s). It is possible, but rare, to have a heart attack without chest pain.
- Difficulty breathing; gasping; shortness of breath
- Sensation of heart palpitations (irregular heartbeat)

The symptoms described above frequently appear with one or more of the following (Figure 74):

- Heavy perspiration
- Sudden dizziness; lightheadedness
- Belching; nausea; vomiting. (Heart attacks are often mistaken for indigestion.)
- Pale or bluish skin and lips
- Cool, clammy skin
- Anxiety; sense of doom
- Shock
- Unconsciousness

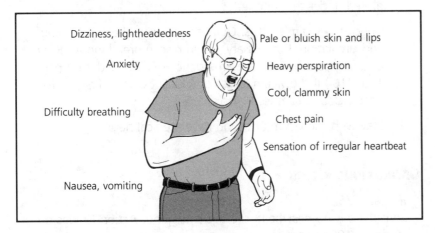

Figure 74
Signs and symptoms of a heart attack. Any or all of these may occur.

Angina attacks often come after physical exertion, emotional stress, exposure to cold, and overeating.

Heart attacks are often associated with old age, smoking, overweight, a sedentary lifestyle, stress, drug use, family history of heart disease, personal history of angina attacks, poor diet, high serum cholesterol levels, high blood pressure, and diabetes. Chest pain that comes on while someone is at rest is a reason for concern, particularly if the person has a history of heart problems.

FIRST AID

Conscious Victim

- Call EMS.
- Notify the victim's physician, if time permits.

DO NOT wait to see if the pain goes away.
DO NOT give the victim anything to eat or drink.
DO NOT give the victim any medication unless it has been prescribed specifically for him or her.
DO NOT allow the victim to exert himself or herself.

1. Calm and reassure the victim.

2. Encourage the victim to rest in a comfortable position. If the victim is having breathing problems, *do not* force him or her to lie down. It is more difficult to breathe when lying down.

3. Loosen any clothing around the victim's neck, chest, and waist.

4. Keep the victim warm.

5. If the victim has prescribed angina medication on hand, help him or her take it. (Usually this is a nitroglycerine tablet that is placed under the tongue.)

6. Check the victim's ABCs. Open the airway; check breathing and circulation. If necessary, begin rescue breathing, CPR, or bleeding control. (See the Emergency Action Guides on pages 199–210.) If the victim loses consciousness, give first aid for an unconscious victim (see next section).

7. Stay with the victim until you have medical help.

FIRST AID

Unconscious Victim

- Call EMS.
- If there is no heartbeat, see the Emergency Action Guides on pages 199–210.
- Check for a medical alert tag.
- Notify the victim's physician, if time permits.

DO NOT leave the victim alone.

Check the victim's ABCs. Open the airway; check breathing and circulation. If necessary, begin rescue breathing, CPR, or bleeding control. (See the Emergency Action Guides on pages 199–210.) Continue until you have medical help.

If the ABCs are present, give first aid for unconsciousness. (See **Un-consciousness** on page 182.) Continue to monitor the victim's ABCs until you have medical help.

More on the Subject

If prescribed angina medication relieves the victim's chest pain within 3 minutes, he or she is probably having an angina attack rather than a true heart attack. However, if the attack recurs, is more severe than usual, or seems "different," it may well be a heart attack. Get medical help immediately.

Your body functions properly within only a limited internal temperature range. If your body's temperature-regulating mechanisms are overwhelmed, your core temperature can skyrocket above a safe level.

A victim of heat illness may start by experiencing muscle cramps. These are brought on by the loss of salt from heavy perspiring. If the victim does not cool off at this point, he or she may develop *heat exhaustion* because of dehydration. The most severe form of heat illness is *heatstroke* (also called sunstroke), which can cause shock, brain damage, and death.

Being in a hot environment — for example, outdoors on a hot and humid day, or inside in a hot, poorly ventilated space — is only one factor that can lead to heat illness. Internal factors are also important. Certain medications, for example, can alter the body's response to heat and sun, and consuming alcohol before or after vigorous exercise may increase the risk of heat illness. Children and older people are more susceptible, and they tend to go from feeling fine to sudden collapse. Even a champion athlete in superb condition can succumb to heat illness if he or she ignores the warning signs.

Signs and Symptoms

Heat Cramps

- Muscle cramps, often in the abdomen or legs
- Heavy perspiration
- Lightheadedness; weakness

Heat Exhaustion

- Cool, pale or red, moist skin. (Even if the victim's internal temperature is rising, his or her skin may still be cool.)
- Dilated (larger than normal) pupils
- Headache
- Extreme thirst
- Nausea; vomiting
- Irrational behavior
- Weakness; dizziness
- Unconsciousness

Heatstroke

- Raised body temperature (above 102° Fahrenheit)
- Dry, hot, red skin
- Dark urine
- Small pupils
- Rapid, weak pulse
- Rapid, shallow breathing
- Extreme confusion
- Weakness
- Seizures
- Unconsciousness

Heat illness is most common in children and older people and in people who are out of shape or obese. It is also associated with the use of alcohol; inappropriate use of drugs; certain medications; dehydration; exposure to heat (indoors or outdoors); and prolonged exertion, especially in children.

FIRST AID

Heat Cramps

- If the victim's condition does not improve, or if it worsens despite treatment, call EMS.

DO NOT underestimate the seriousness of heat illness, especially if the victim is a child, is elderly, or is injured.

DO NOT give the victim liquids that contain alcohol or caffeine. These drugs interfere with the body's ability to regulate its internal temperature.

DO NOT give the victim over-the-counter medications that are used to treat fever (for example, aspirin). They will not be effective, and they may be harmful.

DO NOT give the victim salt tablets. Salt is appropriate, but it should be taken as a salt and water solution.

DO NOT overlook possible complications resulting from the victim's ongoing medical problems (for example, high blood pressure or heart disease).

1. Have the victim rest with his or her feet elevated 8 to 12 inches.

2. Cool the victim. (See box.) *Do not* use an alcohol rub.

3. Give the victim electrolyte beverages to sip (for example, Gatorade or Pedialyte) or make a salted drink by adding 1 teaspoon

How to Cool a Victim of Heat Illness

A victim of heat illness needs help right away. Don't worry about subjecting the victim to extremes in temperature; the important thing is to cool him or her immediately.

Take the victim's temperature as you begin your cooling efforts to see how serious his or her condition is. Take it again after a few minutes to see if it is being brought under control.

To cool the victim, you can use a combination of approaches, depending upon the circumstances:

- Move the victim into the shade, into a cool room, or to an air-conditioned building or car.
- Spray the victim with a hose, or pour a bucket of water over him or her (not in the face). Tell the person what you're going to do, and *do not* use these measures if the victim is confused.
- Wrap the victim in wet towels or sheets, then turn on a fan. Evaporation is a very effective way to cool off.
- Place cold compresses on the victim's neck, groin, and armpits.
- If medical help is not immediately available and you suspect heatstroke, immerse the victim in cold water (bath, lake, stream), but only if you can carefully monitor his or her level of alertness and ABCs (airway, breathing, and circulation).

Once the victim's temperature is down to 100° Fahrenheit, you can ease up on your cooling efforts, but keep checking the victim's temperature every half hour for the next 3 to 4 hours. There is a possibility it may rise again.

of salt to 1 quart of water. Try to give a half cup every 15 minutes. (If electrolyte beverages or salt are not *immediately* available, give the victim cool water.)

4. To relieve muscle cramps, massage the affected muscles gently but firmly until they relax.

FIRST AID

Heat Exhaustion

- If the victim's condition does not improve, or if it worsens despite treatment, call EMS.

DO NOT underestimate the seriousness of heat illness, especially if the victim is a child, is elderly, or is injured.

DO NOT give the victim liquids that contain alcohol or caffeine. These drugs interfere with the body's ability to regulate its internal temperature.

DO NOT give the victim over-the-counter medications that are used to treat fever (for example, aspirin). They will not be effective, and they may be harmful.

DO NOT give the victim salt tablets. Salt is appropriate, but it should be taken as a salt and water solution.

DO NOT overlook possible complications resulting from the victim's ongoing medical problems (for example, high blood pressure or heart disease).

1. Have the victim rest with his or her feet elevated 8 to 12 inches.

2. Cool the victim. (See box on page 157.) *Do not* use an alcohol rub.

3. Give the victim electrolyte beverages to sip (for example, Gatorade or Pedialyte) or make a salted drink by adding 1 teaspoon of salt to 1 quart of water. Try to give a half cup every 15 minutes. (If electrolyte beverages or salt are not *immediately* available, give the victim cool water.)

4. Monitor the victim for signs of shock, including bluish lips and fingernails and decreasing alertness. (See **Shock** on page 172.)

5. If the victim starts having seizures, protect him or her from injury and give first aid for convulsions. (See **Seizures** on page 168.)

6. If the victim loses consciousness, give first aid for unconsciousness. (See **Unconsciousness** on page 182.)

Heat Stroke

- Call EMS.

DO NOT give the victim anything by mouth — not even salted drinks.

DO NOT give the victim over-the-counter medications that are used to treat fever (for example, aspirin). They will not be effective, and they may be harmful.

DO NOT overlook possible complications resulting from the victim's ongoing medical problems (for example, high blood pressure or heart disease).

1. Cool the victim. (See box on page 157.) *Do not* use an alcohol rub.

2. Give first aid for shock. Lay the victim flat and elevate his or her legs 8 to 12 inches. *Do not* place the victim in the shock position if you suspect any head, neck, back, or leg injury; if he or she is having breathing problems; or if the position makes the victim uncomfortable. (See **Shock** on page 172.)

3. If the victim starts having seizures, protect him or her from injury and give first aid for convulsions. (See **Seizures** on page 168.)

4. If the victim loses consciousness, give first aid for unconsciousness. (See **Unconsciousness** on page 182.)

5. Keep the victim cool as you await medical help.

Heimlich Maneuver *See Choking*

Hemorrhage *See Bleeding*

Inhalation Poisoning *See Poison*

Insulin Reaction *See Unconsciousness*

Leg Injury *See Bone, Joint, and Muscle Injuries*

Mouth Injury *See Facial Injury*

Mouth-to-Mouth Resuscitation
See Cardiopulmonary Arrest

Neck Injury *See Spinal Injury*

Nose Injury

The nose has many nerves and blood vessels, which means nose injuries can be bloody and painful. Nose problems also can be frightening because they can make it hard for the victim to breathe freely. Common problems that affect the nose include nosebleeds, an object lodged in a nostril, and broken nasal bones. A severe blow to the nose can cause bleeding into the septum, or wall between the nostrils (a *septal hematoma*). This must be drained by a physician to prevent damage from occurring.

Nose problems are often part of a larger picture. Clear or bloody fluid coming from the nose can indicate serious head injury (see **Head Injury** on page 147). Nose injury and neck injury are often seen together because a blow that is forceful enough to injure the nose may be strong enough to injure the neck. (See **Spinal Injury** on page 175.)

If nose tissue has been torn off, see **Amputation** on page 48.
If the nose is frostbitten, see **Cold Exposure** on page 117.
If the victim has a nosebleed or broken nose and is unconscious, see **Unconsciousness** on page 182. It is important to protect an unconscious victim's airway by putting him or her in a position that allows blood to drain.

Signs and Symptoms

Nosebleeds

- Blood coming from the nostrils
- Bleeding into the back of the throat
- Sensation of fullness in the ears (due to bleeding from the back of the nose)
- Gagging, coughing up blood, or choking (due to bleeding into the throat)

Object Lodged in the Nose

- Irritation; sensation of foreign body in the nostril
- Blood or pus coming from the nose
- Obstructed air flow through the affected nostril

Broken Nose

- Pain
- Swelling
- Bruising around the eyes
- Blood coming from the nose
- Misshapen appearance
- Cuts or other signs of direct trauma

Nosebleeds

Nosebleeds can be the result of trauma to the nose or can occur spontaneously. Many medical conditions, such as bleeding abnormalities, high blood pressure, allergies, or colds, can bring on nosebleeds. Other causes are nosepicking, nasal sprays, strenuous exercise, and very cold or very dry air. Most nosebleeds don't need medical attention, but get medical help if the victim has high blood pressure, is on blood-thinning medication, takes large doses of aspirin, or is known to bleed or bruise easily.

Most nosebleeds come from blood vessels in the front of the nose. Some are caused by bleeding from the back of the nose into the throat (*posterior* bleeding); these are more difficult to control and almost always require medical attention.

- If you suspect neck injury or serious head injury, call EMS.

1. Calm and reassure the victim. Encourage him or her to breathe through the mouth.

FIRST AID

2. Have the victim sit down and lean forward. This will help keep blood from going down the back of his or her throat.

3. Check to see if there is an object in the victim's nose and remove it if necessary (see below).

4. If you can see clots in the nostril, have the victim blow them out. Then pinch the soft part of the victim's nose firmly for a full 15 minutes without releasing. Place a cold compress on the bridge of the nose.

5. If the victim's nose is still bleeding after 15 minutes, repeat this procedure one more time. If the nose is still bleeding after a second attempt, get medical help.

FIRST AID

Object Lodged in the Nose

If an object lodged in the nose is not removed promptly, it may lodge further back in the nose, making removal extremely difficult and possibly causing infection.

DO NOT use tweezers or other instruments to remove an object from the nose.

1. Determine which nostril is affected, but do not have the victim breathe in sharply, since this may force the object further up the nose.

2. Gently press the other nostril with 1 finger.

3. Have the victim blow his or her nose.

4. If the object is still lodged, give the victim some pepper to sniff and encourage him or her to sneeze.

5. If the object is still lodged, get medical help.

FIRST AID

Broken Nose

A broken nose may or may not look misshapen. If you suspect a broken nose, get medical help. Without medical attention, broken nasal bones may heal out of alignment, which can affect the victim's appearance as well as his or her breathing.

- If you suspect neck injury or serious head injury, call EMS.

DO NOT try to straighten a misshapen nose.

1. Calm and reassure the victim. Encourage the victim to breathe through the mouth.

2. Have the victim sit down and lean forward. This will help keep blood from going down the back of the throat.

3. Have the victim apply a cold compress to the nose until you get medical help. (You can apply the compress yourself, but the victim will better know how much pressure to apply.)

More on the Subject

To prevent a recurrence of nosebleed, the victim should avoid physical exertion for 12 hours; touch the nose gently or not at all for 24 hours; avoid blowing the nose for 24 hours; elevate the head with pillows when lying down; sneeze with the mouth open; breathe through the mouth as much as possible; apply moisturizer and use a humidifier at night to help keep the inside of the nose from drying out; and avoid hot beverages, alcoholic beverages, smoking, and aspirin for 1 week.

Overdose *See Drug Abuse*

Poison

A person can be poisoned by ingestion (swallowing), inhalation (breathing in), skin contact, or injection. A poisoning emergency can be life-threatening. The first aid you give before you get medical help can save the victim's life.

In a poisoning emergency, rapid first aid is critical. With ingestion poisoning, your goal is to rid the victim's body of the poison before it has time to be absorbed.

A poisoning victim may not be able to tell you what happened — for example, the victim may be a toddler or be incoherent or unconscious. Sometimes the victim has intentionally taken drugs or chemicals for suicidal or mind-altering purposes and won't volunteer this information unless you ask.

Suspect poisoning if someone suddenly becomes ill for no apparent reason; begins to act in an unusual way; is depressed and suddenly becomes ill; is found near a toxic substance (for example, a chemical, medication, or poisonous plant); may have eaten contaminated or poisonous food or may have drunk contaminated water; has been breathing any unusual fumes; or has stains, liquids, or powders on his or her clothing, skin, or lips. Unintentional overdoses of medications are common, particularly among children.

It's important to note that the absence of a warning on a package label does not necessarily mean the product is safe.

Suspect inhalation poisoning if the victim was near something that burns (furnace, automobile, fire, etc.) in a poorly ventilated area or was working near hazardous materials. Inhalation poisoning can be caused by smoke, carbon dioxide, carbon monoxide (for example, from automobile exhaust or from an improperly functioning furnace), natural gas, ammonia and other chemical fumes, anesthetics, and fumes from paints and solvents. You may not be able to see or smell dangerous fumes or gases.

Signs and symptoms of poisoning can take time to develop. If you suspect that a poisoning has occurred, get medical help right away. Do not wait for symptoms to become obvious.

If the victim has received a venomous bite or sting, see **Bites and Stings** on page 50.

If the victim has inhaled concentrated chemical fumes, he or she may have an airway burn. See **Burns** on page 84.

If the victim has spilled a chemical on himself or herself, see **Chemical Exposure** on page 97.

For a list of commonly ingested poisonous substances, see page 218.

For a list of poisonous plants, see page 259.

Signs and Symptoms

Signs and symptoms of poisoning vary widely and depend upon the type of poisoning that has occurred, the time that has elapsed, and the size and health of the victim. They may be both local (for example, mouth burns) and generalized (for example, a skin rash). They can include:

- Headache; irritability
- Chills
- Increased salivation; pain on swallowing
- Dizziness; weakness; drowsiness
- Pale skin
- Fever
- Depression
- Loss of appetite
- Nausea; abdominal pain; diarrhea; vomiting

- Double vision; blurred vision; visual disturbances; pupils unusually large or small
- Unusual breath odor
- Numbness and dryness of the nose or mouth
- Skin rash; chemical burns on skin
- Chemical burns around the nose and mouth; facial burns; singed nasal hairs
- Bluish lips
- Chest pain; cough; shortness of breath; difficulty breathing
- Heart palpitations
- Muscle twitching
- Loss of bladder or bowel control
- Seizures
- Stupor
- Unconsciousness

Ingestion Poisoning
(Poisoning by Swallowing)

FIRST AID

One form of ingestion poisoning is food poisoning, a general term that covers a variety of conditions. Suspect food poisoning if the victim ate any food that "didn't taste right" or that may have been old, improperly prepared, contaminated, left at room temperature for a long time, or processed with an excessive amount of chemicals. You should also suspect food poisoning if several people who ate together become ill. Water, too, can be contaminated. Often there are no telltale signs that food or water isn't safe. Some exotic foods contain poison and are hazardous if they aren't properly prepared. Certain mushrooms and types of shellfish are poisonous and should never be eaten.

Botulism is a form of food poisoning that can cause paralysis and death if it is not treated. Botulism toxins are most often found in home-canned vegetables, honey, and smoked meats or fish. Signs and symptoms develop within 12 to 36 hours and include headache, dizziness, slurred speech, difficulty swallowing, and difficulty breathing.

- Try to identify the poison. Seek information from the victim or bystanders and look for clues. Save any empty container, spoiled food, or poisonous plant for analysis. Save any vomit and keep it with the victim if he or she is taken to an emergency facility.
- Call your local Poison Control Center for advice. Be prepared to tell them the type of poison, when the poisoning occurred, the victim's age, his or her symptoms, whether or not the victim has

had anything to eat or drink since the poisoning occurred, and how long it would take you to get to the nearest emergency facility.

- If you don't know the correct phone number or have no Poison Control Center in your area, call EMS, the nearest hospital emergency department, or a physician for advice.

DO NOT wait for signs and symptoms to develop if you suspect a poisoning emergency.

DO NOT use any "universal antidote."

DO NOT try to neutralize the poison with vinegar, lemon juice, or any other substance unless you are told to do so by the Poison Control Center or a physician.

DO NOT induce vomiting unless you are told to do so by the Poison Control Center or a physician. A strong poison that burns on the way down will also burn on the way up. Also, petroleum products can cause a severe form of pneumonia if any vomit is inhaled.

DO NOT give an unconscious victim anything by mouth.

DO NOT rely solely on product label information, which may be incorrect.

1. Check the victim's ABCs. Open the airway; check breathing and circulation. If necessary, begin rescue breathing, CPR, or bleeding control. (See the Emergency Action Guides on pages 199–210.)

   If the ABCs are present but the victim is unconscious, place him or her in the recovery position (see page 183) and continue to monitor his or her ABCs.

   If the ABCs are present and the victim is conscious, have him or her assume the recovery position. Continue to monitor ABCs.

2. If the victim starts having seizures, protect him or her from injury and give first aid for convulsions. (See **Seizures** on page 168.)

3. If the victim throws up, protect the airway. (See Vomiting on page 151.) If you must clear the victim's airway, wrap a cloth around your fingers before cleaning out his or her mouth and throat.

4. Calm and reassure the victim and keep him or her comfortable while you wait for medical help.

How to Rescue a Victim of Possible Inhalation Poisoning

Inhalation poisoning most often occurs within an enclosed, poorly ventilated space. If someone has been overcome by smoke, fumes, or gas, he or she needs fresh air immediately.

If you decide to enter the area:

- Call for EMS. Attract the attention of bystanders. *Never* attempt a rescue without notifying others.
- Check to see if protective breathing gear is available. If it isn't, place a wet cloth over your nose and mouth.
- If possible, open windows and doors to help disperse the fumes.
- Do not light a match, flip a switch, or produce any flame or spark. Some gases can ignite.
- Take several deep breaths of fresh air, then hold your breath as you go in.

As you rescue the victim:

- Stay below smoke or fumes that are visible in the upper part of the room. Keep your head above exhaust or heavy fumes that are near the floor.
- If possible, quickly shut off any open source of fumes.
- Do not start any first aid until you and the victim are in fresh air.
- Use the clothes drag technique (see page 178) to immediately remove the victim from the area.

Once you and the victim are in fresh air, begin first aid for inhalation poisoning.

Inhalation Poisoning
(Poisoning by Breathing)

- Rescue the victim from the smoke, gas, or fumes (see box).
- Call your local Poison Control Center for advice. Be prepared to tell them what the victim inhaled, when the poisoning occurred, the victim's age, his or her signs and symptoms, and how long it would take you to get to the nearest emergency facility.
- If you don't know the correct phone number or have no Poison Control Center in your area, call EMS, the nearest hospital emergency department, or a physician.

DO NOT wait for signs and symptoms to develop if you suspect inhalation poisoning may have occurred.

FIRST AID

DO NOT give an unconscious victim anything by mouth.

DO NOT rely on product label information, which may be incorrect.

1. Check the victim's ABCs. Open the airway; check breathing and circulation. If necessary, begin rescue breathing, CPR, or bleeding control. (See the Emergency Action Guides on pages 199–210.)

    If the ABCs are present but the victim is unconscious, place him or her in the recovery position (see page 183) and continue to monitor his or her ABCs.

    If the ABCs are present and the victim is conscious, have him or her rest in the recovery position. Continue to monitor the victim's ABCs.

2. Check the victim's eyes and skin for chemical burns. If there are any, flush the affected area(s) thoroughly with cold water for 15 minutes. (See **Eye Injury** on page 136 and **Chemical Exposure** on page 97.)

3. If the victim starts having seizures, protect him or her from injury and see **Seizures** below.

4. If the victim throws up, protect his or her airway. (See Vomiting on page 151.)

5. Get medical help, even if the victim seems completely recovered.

Rescue Breathing *See Cardiopulmonary Arrest*

Seizures

A *seizure* is a sudden involuntary muscle contraction, usually due to uncontrolled electrical activity in the brain. Many different problems — some more serious than others — can cause brain cells to fire abnormally.

In some cases, an individual can sense that a seizure is going to occur. He or she may hallucinate, hear an imagined sound, get a strange taste in the mouth, experience abdominal pain, or feel an urgent need to get to safety.

Most seizures last from 30 to 45 seconds. Seizures are also known as *convulsions*. Seizures associated with fever are called *febrile seizures*. (See box on page 170.) When seizures recur, and there are no underlying causes that can be treated directly, a person is said to have *epilepsy*. Epilepsy is usually well controlled with medication.

There is nothing you can do to stop seizures once they have started. First aid is aimed at protecting the victim from injury and getting medical help as needed.

If a toddler experiences multiple seizures for the first time, assume he or she has swallowed poison. See **Poison** on page 163.

Signs and Symptoms

- Local tingling or twitching in one part of the body ("focal seizure")
- Brief blackout or period of confused behavior ("petit mal" seizure)
- Sudden falling; loss of consciousness
- Drooling; frothing at the mouth
- Vigorous muscle spasms; twitching; jerking limbs; stiffening ("grand mal" seizures)
- Grunting; snorting
- Loss of bladder or bowel control
- Temporary cessation of breathing

Seizures are often associated with epilepsy; high blood pressure; heart disease; brain tumor, stroke, or other brain illness or injury; shaking young children violently; fever in children (see box on page 170); head injury; electric shock; heat illness; poisoning; venomous bites and stings; choking; and drug or alcohol overdose or withdrawal.

Seizures

- Check to see if the victim has a medical alert tag.
- Call EMS if the victim:
  - Has continuous or recurring seizures (more than 1 episode per hour)
  - Does not awaken between seizures
  - Is ill or injured
  - Has never had seizures before
  - Has diabetes or high blood pressure
  - Is pregnant
  - Has seizures that last longer than 2 minutes
  - Had a seizure in the water
  - Seems weak and feverish after the seizures have stopped

FIRST AID

Fever

An oral temperature of over 99.4° Fahrenheit or a rectal temperature of over 100.4° Fahrenheit is considered fever. Fever is one of the body's responses to illness or injury. Elevated temperature can also result from heat exposure. (See **Heat Illnesses** on page 155.)

Febrile Seizures

A high temperature does not necessarily mean the victim is seriously ill. Some children, however, have febrile seizures when a high fever is rising or falling. Although they are extremely frightening for the parent or caregiver, these seizures usually are self-limited and pass relatively quickly.

After an episode of febrile seizures, take the child's temperature. It is important to bring the child's temperature to normal. Remove any clothes and bedclothes, give the child a sponge bath on a counter with lukewarm water, and turn on a fan. Stop if the child shivers. (Do not place the child in a bathtub because he or she could have another seizure in the water.) The child's physician may recommend an over-the-counter medication such as acetaminophen or ibuprofen. Notify the child's physician that a seizure has occurred. If the cause of the seizure is unknown, ask a physician to determine if it was caused by infection.

When to Get Medical Help for Fever

Fever is not always cause for alarm, but sometimes it is a sign of a serious problem. Seek immediate medical attention if:

- Fever is over 100.2° Fahrenheit (measured rectally) in a baby under 3 months of age or over 101° in a baby 3 to 6 months of age
- Fever is over 103° Fahrenheit
- Fever of over 101° Fahrenheit (measured rectally) lasts more than 24 hours
- Fever is accompanied by:

  Difficulty breathing
  Unusual skin color (blue, gray, purple)
  A rash of tiny red or purple dots under the skin
  Shock
  Stiff neck
  Bulging fontanel (soft spot on baby's skull)
  Signs of dehydration (sunken fontanel, little or no urine, dry
     mouth, sunken eyeballs, severe thirst, sleepiness, weakness)

If the victim appears to be very ill, take steps to reduce the fever while you seek medical assistance. Don't hesitate to call a physician if you are unsure whether or not the fever needs to be evaluated.

- Try to time the duration of the seizures so you'll have a measurement of how severe they are.

DO NOT restrain the victim.

DO NOT place anything between the victim's teeth during a seizure (including your fingers).

DO NOT move the victim unless he or she is in danger or near something hazardous (for example, stairs or sharp-edged furniture).

DO NOT try to make the victim "snap out of it." He or she can't.

DO NOT perform rescue breathing on a seizure victim, even if he or she is turning blue. Most seizures end long before brain damage would begin.

DO NOT give the victim anything by mouth until the seizures have stopped and the victim is fully awake and alert.

1. If you are there when the victim feels an episode coming on or starts to fall, try to protect him or her from falling. Lay the victim on the ground or on the floor in a safe area.

2. Remove any hard or sharp objects from the area. Clear away furniture, if possible, and cushion the area with pillows or blankets.

3. Loosen any tight clothing, particularly around the victim's neck.

4. After the seizures stop:

   - *If you do not suspect spinal injury,* place the victim in the recovery position (see page 183) so fluids can drain.
   - *If you do suspect spinal injury,* log-roll the victim onto his or her side, supporting the head and neck (see page 177). This is best accomplished with the assistance of several bystanders.

5. If the victim throws up, take steps to protect the airway. (See Vomiting on page 151.)

6. Most seizure victims regain consciousness but then go into a deep sleep. *Do not* try to prevent the victim from sleeping after the seizures have passed.

   Someone with a history of seizures may take up to an hour to recover after a seizure. The usual recovery sequence after a grand mal seizure (in which the victim loses consciousness) is: seizures stop; victim goes into a deep sleep; victim awakens but is disoriented; victim starts to remember personal information; victim starts to remember general information.

7. Monitor the victim carefully while he or she recovers. Check his or her ABCs and watch for recurring seizures.

8. If the seizures were associated with fever, take steps to bring the fever down (see box on page 170).

9. If the victim neglected to take prescribed seizure medication, help the victim take it after he or she recovers.

10. Stay with the victim until he or she fully regains consciousness or until you have medical help.

Shock

Shock can occur when something happens that reduces the flow of blood throughout the body, limiting the amount of oxygen the blood carries to the body's cells. It's a life-threatening condition that requires immediate medical treatment. Preventing shock is easier than trying to treat it once it happens. By giving first aid early, you can help keep shock from getting worse.

Shock has many causes, and some degree of shock can accompany any medical emergency. When a victim has gone into shock, it is important to give first aid for the underlying illness or injury. Any problem that causes a reduced rate of blood flow (for example, heart failure) or a reduction in blood volume (for example, dehydration or severe bleeding) can lead to shock. Conditions that stress the body, including heat or cold, can also cause shock. In some people, emotional distress can produce a condition that mimics shock.

Shock can worsen rapidly. Stay alert for changes in the victim's level of consciousness as well as the nature of his or her pulse. A pulse that becomes fainter or faster is a sign of distress. Be prepared to begin rescue breathing or CPR as needed.

If signs of shock are accompanied by signs of severe allergic reaction (*anaphylactic shock*) — including weakness, nausea, difficulty breathing or swallowing, swelling of the face or tongue, hives, flushed face — see **Allergic Reaction** on page 45.
If the victim has low blood sugar (*insulin shock*), see **Unconsciousness** on page 182.

Signs and Symptoms

- Weakness; dizziness
- Restlessness; anxiety; confusion
- Decreasing alertness
- Cold, clammy skin
- Extreme paleness
- Bluish lips and fingernails
- Chest pain
- Rapid, shallow breathing
- Numbness; paralysis
- Nausea; vomiting
- Intense thirst
- Unconsciousness

Shock is often associated with burns, drug overdose, electrical injury, heart attack, heatstroke, low blood sugar, hypothermia, over-whelming infection (*septic shock*), poisoning, severe allergic reaction, severe bleeding, severe vomiting and/or diarrhea, and spinal injury.

Shock Victim with No Spinal Injury

FIRST AID

- Call EMS.
- Try to determine the cause of shock. Check the victim for a medical alert tag.

DO NOT give the victim anything by mouth.

1. Check the victim's ABCs. Open the airway; check breathing and circulation. If necessary, begin rescue breathing, CPR, or bleeding control. (See the Emergency Action Guides on pages 199–210.)
2. Place the victim in the shock position (Figure 75). Lay the victim flat and elevate the feet 8 to 12 inches, using any available

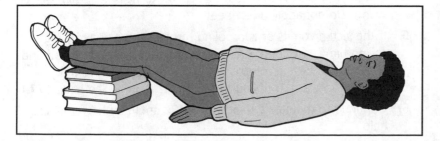

Figure 75
The shock position

support. *Do not* place pillows under the victim's head, and *do not* use the shock position if you suspect the victim has any head, neck, back, or leg injury; if the victim is having breathing problems; or if the position makes the victim uncomfortable. If the victim has received a venomous bite, *do not* raise the bite above the level of the victim's heart.

3. Give first aid for the underlying illness or injury.

4. Keep the victim comfortable. Loosen any constricting clothing and cover him or her with a coat or blanket to help keep him or her warm. *Do not* apply direct heat.

5. If the victim vomits or is drooling, turn the head to one side so fluids can drain.

6. Continue to monitor the victim's ABCs until you have medical help.

FIRST AID

Shock Victim with Possible Spinal Injury

Do not move a victim who you suspect has a neck or back injury unless he or she is in immediate danger. (See How to Move a Victim with a Suspected Spinal Injury on page 178.) If you are not sure whether the victim has a spinal injury, assume he or she does.

- Call EMS.
- Try to determine the cause of shock. Check the victim for a medical alert tag.

DO NOT give the victim anything by mouth.

1. Check the victim's ABCs. Open the airway; check breathing and circulation. If necessary, begin rescue breathing, CPR, or bleeding control. (See the Emergency Action Guides on pages 199–210.)

2. Keep the victim in the position you found him or her. *Do not* place the victim in the shock position.

3. Give first aid for the underlying illness or injury.

4. Cover the victim with a coat or blanket to help keep him or her warm. *Do not* apply direct heat.

5. If the victim vomits or is drooling, protect the airway by log-rolling him or her onto one side while supporting the head and neck. This is best accomplished with the help of several bystanders to assist in rolling the victim as a unit. (See page 177.)

6. Continue to monitor the victim's ABCs until you have medical help.

If You Suspect a Head, Neck, or Back Injury

If you think the victim might have a head, neck, or back injury, you will have to take that into account as you open the airway. Simply lift the chin rather than tilt the head back. If you cannot breathe air into the victim, then try tilting the head back very slightly.

Your *spine* is an exquisitely designed structure made up of a column of *vertebrae* (curving bones) with disks of cartilage between them. The vertebrae are bound together by flexible ligaments and are attached to layer upon layer of muscles. The spine extends from the base of your skull to the end of your tailbone and supports your skull, ribs, shoulder bones, and pelvis. It also protects the *spinal cord*, a cylinder of nerve tissue that runs through a channel in the center of the vertebrae. The spinal cord transmits nerve impulses to and from the brain and controls the body (Figure 76).

Spinal injury can involve some or all parts of the neck and back — muscles, ligaments, bones, and nerves. It's possible to injure your vertebrae without harming your spinal cord.

The spinal cord is connected to networks of nerves that branch out into the trunk, arms, and legs. Damage to the spinal cord is extremely

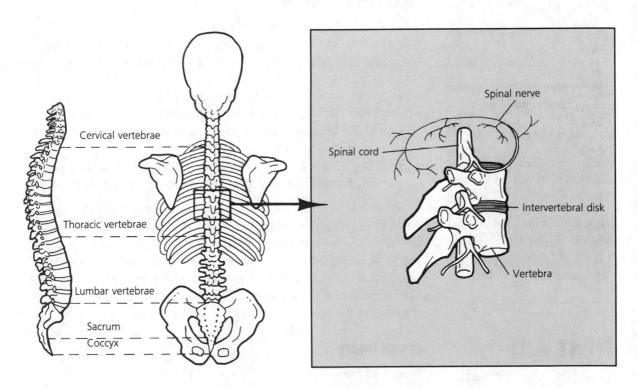

Figure 76
Anatomy of the spine

serious because it can mean the loss of sensation and function in the parts of the body below the site of the injury.

When someone has a spinal injury, additional movement may cause further damage to the spine or spinal cord. For example, a broken vertebra may cut or crush the spinal cord, causing shock, permanent paralysis or disability, or even death. The purpose of first aid is to prevent further harm to the victim until you have medical help. *Do not* move the victim unless he or she is in urgent danger. If you must move the victim without the help of emergency personnel, it is vital that you take steps to prevent any twisting or bending of the victim's body (see box on page 178).

If you come upon an unconscious person and are unsure whether or not spinal injury has occurred, *assume it has.* Obvious injuries to the face, neck, or back all suggest possible spinal injury. So does evidence that the victim has fallen or been thrown some distance. The signs and symptoms of spinal cord injury almost always appear immediately.

Signs and Symptoms

- Pain in the head, neck, or back
- Pain in the abdomen and back. (The degree of pain may not tell you how severe the injury is because individual tolerance for pain varies.)
- Numbness or tingling down an arm or leg
- Weakness, loss of sensation, or paralysis in arms or legs
- Inability to move parts of the body at will
- Loss of bladder or bowel control
- Shock. (Signs and symptoms include pale, clammy skin; weakness; bluish lips and fingernails; and decreasing alertness.)

Spinal injuries often result from direct trauma to the face, neck, or back; direct trauma to the spine (bullet, stab wound); diving accidents; falls from high places; exertion; extra weight; sudden movements; twisting, awkward positions; high heels; and stressing the muscles on one side of the back more than the muscles on the other side. Victims of electric shock or explosions often suffer spinal injury from being thrown to the ground.

Spinal Injury

- Call EMS.
- Keep the victim absolutely still. Unless there is urgent danger, keep the victim in the position found.

If You Suspect a Head, Neck, or Back Injury

If you think the victim might have a head, neck, or back injury, you will have to take that into account as you open the airway. Simply lift the chin rather than tilt the head back. If you cannot breathe air into the victim, then try tilting the head back very slightly.

FIRST AID

- Try to determine what happened.
- Treat any obvious injuries where the victim lies.

DO NOT move the victim unless there is immediate danger.
DO NOT change the victim's position or pick up the victim unless absolutely necessary.
DO NOT twist or bend the victim's head, neck, or back.

1. Check the victim's ABCs. Open the airway; check breathing and circulation. If necessary, begin rescue breathing, CPR, or bleeding control. (See the Emergency Action Guides on pages 199–210.) You may have to roll the victim onto his or her back to begin rescue breathing or CPR. Try to keep the victim's head, neck, and back in line and to roll him or her as a unit. This is best accomplished with the help of several bystanders.

   If the ABCs are present but the victim is unconscious, immobilize the victim's head and neck by placing your hands on both sides of the head (Figure 77). Wait for assistance.

   If the ABCs are present and the victim is conscious, do not allow the victim to move, even if he or she is in a car. (See box on page 180.) Immobilize the victim in the exact position found using towels, blankets, clothing, or any other supporting objects. Then use heavy objects such as books, stones, or baggage to keep those supports in place. Reassure the victim as you wait for emergency personnel.

2. If the victim vomits or is choking on blood, protect his or her airway by log-rolling him or her onto one side. This is best accomplished with the help of several bystanders (Figure 78), but if necessary can be done by one rescuer (Figure 79). Vomiting can indicate internal injuries. (See Vomiting on page 151.)

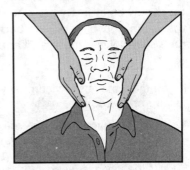

Figure 77
Immobilizing the head and neck

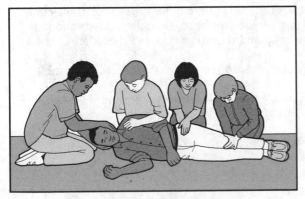

Figure 78   Log roll with several bystanders

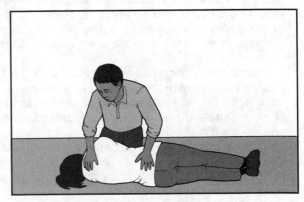

Figure 79   Single rescuer log-roll

Spinal Injury   177

How to Move a Victim with a Suspected Spinal Injury

Never move anyone who could possibly have injured his or her neck or back (spine) unless the scene is unsafe.

It is always best to allow EMS professionals to move a victim with a possible spinal injury. However, there may be a time when you *must* move the victim from an unsafe area. If so, remember to keep the victim's head, neck, and back immobile and his or her body straight. Never twist or bend the victim's spine. Never move a victim sideways to safety.

Immediate Rescue with One Rescuer

If you must move the victim by yourself, you can use the *clothes drag technique* with the victim lying faceup or facedown.

1. Which technique you use will depend in part upon the position in which the victim is lying.
   If the victim is lying sideways, place him or her faceup, remembering to move the body as a unit.
   If the victim already is lying faceup, gently straighten his or her legs.
   If the victim is lying facedown, use the facedown clothes drag technique.
2. Bend your knees and position yourself so you do not have to twist any part of your body awkwardly as you pull the victim.
3. Immobilize the victim's head between your forearms and grab the victim's clothes at his or her shoulders (Figures 80 and 81). If the victim is wearing a jacket, unbutton it to prevent choking.
4. Do not use only the muscles in your back to pull. Instead, use the large muscles of your thighs and abdomen.
5. Walking backward, drag the victim slowly and smoothly to safety.

Immediate Rescue with More Than One Rescuer

If possible, recruit others to help you move the victim. At least four rescuers is ideal. You will also need a board or other rigid surface on which to place the victim. If you have no board, use the rescuers' hands for support.

1. How you proceed depends upon the position of the victim's body.
   If the victim is not lying flat, place a board or other rigid surface that can be lifted (for example, a door) parallel to the victim and at a slight angle. Then log-roll the victim until his or her back touches the board, and gently lower the board to the ground (Figure 82). Be sure to roll the victim as a unit, never twisting or bending the spine. Support the victim's head, shoulders, waist, and legs. If only two rescuers are on hand, have one hold the head and the other hold the shoulders of the victim.
   If the victim is lying flat on his or her back, lift the victim onto the board as carefully as possible, making sure one person supports his or her head.
2. Immobilize the victim's head and neck by wrapping a pillow, blanket, or towel around the head and neck and securing it in place (Figures 83a and 83b). If you have none of these supplies, use your hands (Figure 84).
3. To keep from twisting the upper body, immobilize the victim's arms next to his or her trunk. Bind the victim to the board.
4. As you lift and move the victim, keep everything in line as much as possible so there is no further movement of the victim's head, neck, or back.

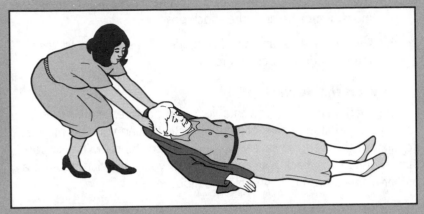

Figure 80
Clothes drag when victim is faceup

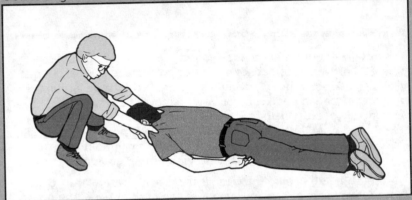

Figure 81
Clothes drag when victim is facedown

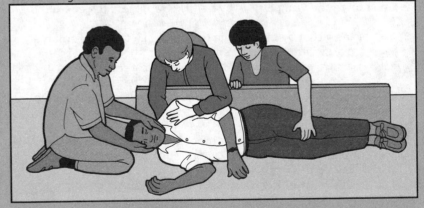

Figure 82
Log-rolling the victim onto a board

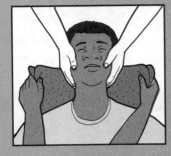

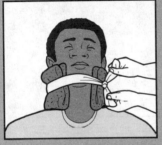

Figure 83 a, b
Immobilizing the head and neck

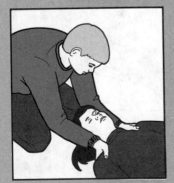

Figure 84
Immobilizing the head and neck with hands only

Spinal Injury   179

3. Keep the victim warm to help prevent shock, but *do not* move him or her into the shock position.

4. Give first aid for any obvious injuries, remembering to keep the victim in the position found.

More on the Subject

Many back injuries are preventable. Good posture, regular exercise, staying fit, and lifting heavy objects correctly (letting your leg muscles do most of the work) all save wear and tear on the back. It is important to discuss any back pain you have with your physician because a proper diagnosis can help you avoid serious injury.

Rescue from an Automobile

It is usually not necessary to move a victim from an automobile before EMS arrives; automobiles do not often explode after accidents. If you can do so without moving the victim, turn off the ignition and set the parking brake. If you *must* remove the victim from an automobile because he or she is in immediate danger, first immobilize the neck and back with a board. If you have no board, you will have to weigh the urgency of moving the victim without a board against waiting for professional help with proper equipment.

1. Insert a board behind the victim's back, being careful not to cause any unnecessary movement of the neck or back. The board should extend from the victim's head to below his or her buttocks (Figure 85).
2. Immobilize the victim's neck by gently wrapping a towel around it.
3. Secure the victim by binding him or her firmly to the board in at least 4 places: around the forehead, around the neck (over the towel), under the armpits, and around the lower abdomen. If possible, secure the victim's arms to the board as well.
4. Tie the victim's knees and ankles together. This will help prevent twisting of the body as you remove the victim from the automobile.
5. Remove the victim from the automobile, being careful not to twist or bend his or her body. Do not pull on the backboard, as this will cause the victim to slip off.

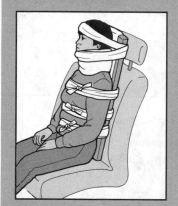

Figure 85
Immobilizing the neck and back in a car

Sports Injuries   *See Bone, Joint, and Muscle Injuries*

Sprains and Strains   *See Bone, Joint, and Muscle Injuries*

When a blood vessel to or within the brain bursts or becomes narrowed by a clot, brain cells in the affected area will begin to die from lack of oxygen. Recognizing the signals and getting immediate medical care can greatly improve the chance of recovery.

A passing loss of function and weakness, including slurred speech, that lasts less than 24 hours may be a passing stroke called a TIA (transient ischemic attack).

Signs and Symptoms

Signs and symptoms of a stroke vary according to the location and size of the blood vessel. One or more of the following may occur:

- Unexplained dizziness or unsteadiness
- Severe headache
- Sudden temporary weakness or numbness of the face, arm, or leg on one side of the body
- Temporary loss of speech; trouble speaking; speech that is difficult to understand
- Temporary vision disturbance
- Unconsciousness

Stroke

FIRST AID

If you suspect a stroke:

1. Check the victim's ABCs. Open the airway; check breathing and circulation. If necessary, begin rescue breathing, CPR, or bleeding control. (See the Emergency Action Guides on pages 199–210.)

2. Have the victim rest in a comfortable position.

3. Call EMS.

4. Do not give the victim anything by mouth.

5. If the victim loses consciousness, place him or her in the recovery position and administer first aid for unconsciousness. (See **Unconsciousness** below.)

6. Continue to monitor the victim's ABCs.

7. Stay with the victim until you have medical help.

Substance Abuse *See Drug Abuse*

Tooth Injury *See Facial Injury*

Unconsciousness

Unconsciousness is an abnormal state in which the victim is not alert and is not fully responsive to his or her surroundings. There are different levels of unconsciousness, ranging from drowsiness to collapse. Someone who is unconscious can be either restless or motionless. Unconsciousness may be brief and light, as in fainting, or profound and prolonged, as in a coma.

Being unconscious is not the same as being asleep. It is difficult or impossible to rouse someone who is unconscious. Unconscious victims can choke to death because they cannot cough, clear their throat, or turn their head if their airway becomes obstructed. First aid is aimed at protecting a victim's airway until the victim revives or gets medical help.

Virtually every major illness or injury can lead to loss of consciousness. Sometimes a blow or a fall can cause internal bleeding, which in time can lead to loss of consciousness. If you come upon someone who is unconscious, assume that he or she is seriously ill or injured. Try to give first aid for the underlying problem. Even if the victim regains consciousness and seems fully recovered, a medical examination is needed to rule out any serious underlying problem.

Following are instructions for first aid for Fainting, Diabetic Emergency, and Unconsciousness. Check for a medical alert tag. If the cause is unknown, give first aid for Unconsciousness.

Signs and Symptoms

An unconscious victim may be:

- Drowsy; disoriented; slipping in and out of consciousness
- In a stupor; incoherent when roused
- In a coma; motionless; silent

How to Place a Victim in the Recovery Position

The recovery position is the safest position for a victim who is unconscious but breathing. This position promotes good circulation and protects the victim's airway by allowing fluids (blood, vomit, etc.) to drain.

The recovery position is not *appropriate if the victim has been seriously injured or if spinal injury is suspected.*

1. Position the victim so he or she is lying faceup.
2. Turn the victim's face toward you.
3. Put the victim's arm (the one nearer you) at the victim's side and place it under the buttock.
4. Place the victim's other arm across his or her chest.
5. Move the victim's far leg over the near leg (Figure 86a) so his or her ankles are crossed.
6. Supporting the victim's head with one hand, grab the clothing at his or her hip and pull him or her toward you (Figure 86b). He or she will roll over.
7. Bend the victim's top arm to support the upper body. Bend the victim's top knee to support the lower body.
8. Gently tilt the victim's head back to make sure his or her airway is open. Air should move freely in and out of his or her mouth.

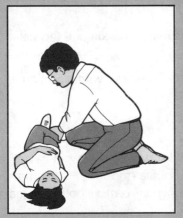
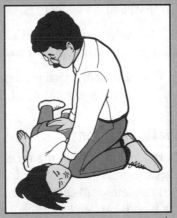
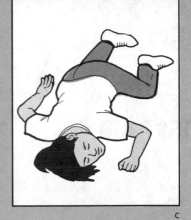

a   b   c

Figure 86 a, b, c
Placing the victim in the recovery position

Fainting

Fainting is a sudden, brief loss of consciousness. Fainting is often caused by low blood sugar or standing in one place for a long time, but there may also be a more serious reason. A brief period of unconsciousness after a head injury is called a *concussion* and is not the same as a fainting spell (see **Head Injury** on page 147).

FIRST AID

Fainting can occur suddenly, or the victim may experience warning signs such as dizziness, nausea, weakness, or blurred vision.

- If the victim does not regain consciousness promptly, call EMS.

DO NOT leave the victim alone.
DO NOT give an unconscious victim anything by mouth.

1. If you see that someone is about to faint, act quickly to prevent him or her from falling. If possible, have the victim lie down.

2. If the victim has fainted, lay him or her faceup on the floor or ground. Elevate the victim's feet 8 to 12 inches to help promote blood circulation to the brain. *Do not* place a pillow under the victim's head; this can block the airway.

3. Loosen the victim's clothing and wipe his or her forehead with cool water. *Do not* try to wake the victim by throwing water on his or her face or by slapping or shaking.

4. If the victim vomits, quickly put him or her in the recovery position (see box on page 183) to protect his or her airway. (See Vomiting on page 151.)

5. As the victim revives, offer reassurance. Discourage the victim from standing up right away.

6. Call EMS if the victim does not fully recover within 5 minutes, is elderly, or complains of illness.

FIRST AID

Diabetic Emergency

Diabetes is a disorder that affects blood sugar. Diabetes can cause unconsciousness in two ways: *hyperglycemia* (too much sugar in the blood) can lead to diabetic coma, and *hypoglycemia* (too little sugar in the blood) can lead to insulin shock.

A diabetic emergency can be difficult to recognize. The victim may appear to be drunk or high or may seem to have suffered a stroke. Check the victim for a medical alert tag.

It can be hard to tell whether the victim is hyperglycemic or hypoglycemic. Hyperglycemia develops gradually and is characterized by thirst, frequent urination, vomiting, flushed skin, rapid breathing, "fruity" breath, and confused or combative behavior. Hypoglycemia progresses more rapidly and is characterized by hunger, pale skin, sweating, poor coordination, disoriented or angry behavior, and, possibly, by seizures.

DO NOT leave the victim alone.

DO NOT give an unconscious victim anything by mouth.

DO NOT try to wake an unconscious victim by throwing water in his or her face or by slapping or shaking.

DO NOT place a pillow under the head of an unconscious victim. This can block the airway.

- If the victim tells you he or she has *high blood sugar*, get medical help immediately. (If the victim is *not sure*, see below.) The victim will need an injection of insulin. If the victim's insulin is on hand, help the victim with his or her medication. If the victim is conscious and can swallow, have him or her drink *unsweetened* fluids to combat dehydration while you wait for medical help.
- If the victim tells you he or she has *low blood sugar* and the victim is *conscious* and can swallow, have him or her eat or drink something sweet (fruit juice, banana, candy, sugar cube). (If the victim is *not sure*, see below.) His or her condition should improve dramatically within 10 minutes. If it does not, get medical help.
- If the victim is *unconscious*, call EMS.
- If the victim is *conscious* and is *not sure* whether the problem is high or low blood sugar, give the victim something sweet while you wait for medical help. If the problem is in fact low blood sugar, the victim's condition will quickly improve. If the problem is high blood sugar, the extra sugar will not significantly affect the victim's condition.

Unconsciousness

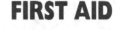

- Try to determine what happened. Check the victim for a medical alert tag.
- If you *cannot* determine why the victim is unconscious, give first aid for unconsciousness until the victim revives. If the victim does not regain consciousness promptly, call EMS.
- If you *can* determine why the victim is unconscious, call EMS. Then give first aid for that specific illness or injury, remembering to protect the victim's airway according to the steps below.

DO NOT leave the victim alone.

DO NOT give an unconscious victim anything by mouth. If the victim revives, *do not* give him or her anything to eat or drink without first consulting a physician.

DO NOT try to wake an unconscious person by throwing water in his or her face or by slapping or shaking.

DO NOT place a pillow under the head of an unconscious victim. This can block the airway.

1. Check the victim's ABCs. Open the airway; check breathing and circulation. If necessary, begin rescue breathing, CPR, or bleeding control. (See the Emergency Action Guides on pages 199–210.)

    If the ABCs are present but the victim is unconscious, be prepared to begin rescue breathing or CPR if the victim's condition worsens. If the victim is having trouble breathing, open the airway. (See the Emergency Action Guides on pages 199–210.)

2. Try to determine whether or not the victim may have injured his or her neck or back.

    If you do not suspect spinal injury, place the victim in the recovery position (see box on page 183).

    If you do suspect spinal injury, leave the victim as found as long as he or she is breathing freely. If the victim starts to choke or vomit, log-roll him or her onto one side, supporting the head and neck (see page 177). This is best accomplished with the help of several bystanders.

3. If the victim becomes restless, gently restrain him or her.

4. If the victim starts having seizures, see **Seizures** on page 168.

5. Keep the victim warm until you have medical help.

Wounds

An *open wound* is an injury that breaks the skin. It can be as shallow as a paper cut or as deep as a gunshot wound.

All wounds need attention in order to prevent infection and promote healing. Get medical help if you cannot stop the bleeding; if the wound is due to an animal or human bite; if the wound is deep, ragged, gaping, or you think it requires stitches; if you cannot get the wound completely clean; if the wound affects a joint or the fingers or toes; if the wound is small but the victim's pain is severe; if the victim has any loss of function or sensation beyond the wound; if the wound is on the face or in another area where there is concern about scarring; or if the victim's immunization against tetanus is not up to date (see box on page 188).

Internal injury is difficult to gauge and can be far more serious than it appears on the surface. In certain parts of the body, important nerves, blood vessels, tendons, and ligaments lie quite close to the skin. A cut to the neck can be fatal if it severs an artery; a cut to the hand can cause loss of function in the fingers if a tendon is severed.

When giving first aid for open wounds, it is important to take health precautions against the transmission of disease. It is best to wear sterile gloves. If you have no gloves, use several layers of dressings or add a layer of plastic wrap between you and the wound. Always wash your hands before and after giving first aid. (For more information on the transmission of infectious diseases, see Health Precautions and Guidelines for the Rescuer on page 25.)

Wounds often become infected. Good circulation promotes healing, and so the farther a wound is from the heart, the longer it takes to heal and the greater the chance of infection. People with diabetes or circulatory problems and older people heal more slowly, so their wounds are also more likely to become infected. Wounds that are at high risk for infection include bites, puncture wounds, foot wounds, crush injuries, wounds that are dirty, and wounds that do not receive prompt medical help.

If any tissue or body part has been crushed or torn off, see **Amputation** on page 48.

If the victim was bitten by a venomous snake, see **Bites and Stings** on page 50.

If a wound is bleeding severely, see **Bleeding** on page 62.

If the victim has a closed wound (one that does not break the skin) or you suspect internal bleeding, see **Bleeding** on page 62.

If the victim has an open wound and you suspect a broken bone, see **Bone, Joint, and Muscle Injuries** on page 69.

If the victim has a chest wound, see **Breathing Problems** on page 79.

If the victim has a serious head injury, see **Head Injury** on page 147.

If applicable, see **Ear Injury** on page 129, **Eye Injury** on page 136, **Facial Injury** on page 142, and **Genital Injury** on page 146.

Signs and Symptoms

- Pain
- Obvious cut, scrape, tear, or puncture
- Bleeding. (The amount of blood is not a good way to judge the severity of the wound.)
- Loss of function farther down from the wound. (A tendon may be severed.)
- Loss of sensation farther down from the wound. (A nerve may be severed.)

Tetanus

Tetanus is an extremely serious disease. Tetanus bacteria are found all over the world in soil, in the air, or on human skin. If these bacteria get into a wound that receives little oxygen (for example, a puncture wound), they can multiply and produce a toxin that affects the central nervous system, leading to muscle spasms and possibly death. A common symptom of tetanus is a stiff jaw (lockjaw).

Wounds that are shallow, clean, have straight edges, and are cared for promptly carry a low risk of tetanus. Wounds that are deep, jagged, dirty, or have gone untreated for several hours carry a high risk of tetanus.

Fortunately, there is a vaccination against tetanus. In the United States the DPT vaccination — which provides immunization against diphtheria, pertussis (whooping cough), and tetanus — is given routinely in childhood. However, tetanus immunity is not permanent. Tetanus boosters are needed every 5 to 10 years. Whether or not someone with a wound should be given the tetanus booster depends upon the wound and the status of the victim's tetanus immunization. Anyone with a wound who has never been immunized against tetanus should be given a tetanus vaccine and booster as soon as possible. A victim who was once immunized but has not received a tetanus booster within the last 10 years should receive one. If it's been over 5 years and the wound is considered high risk, a booster should be given. A tetanus immunization is only effective if given within 72 hours of a wound. Schools and certain jobs require current immunization; check with your physician if you're unsure whether you are current.

Splinters

Splinters must be removed. Do not let a wooden splinter get wet, since this will make it swell, making removal more difficult. Get medical help for large or deep splinters.

1. Wash your hands.

2. Sterilize tweezers and a needle in boiling water or over an open flame, or pour antiseptic solution over them.

3. Try to grab the splinter with the tweezers. Pull the splinter out at the same angle it went in. If the splinter is under a fingernail, you may have to cut a V-shaped notch in the nail in order to get to it.

4. If you cannot grab the splinter with tweezers because it is just under the surface of the skin, use the tip of the needle to lift the splinter out.

5. After all of the splinter is out, wash the area and bandage it. Don't keep trying to remove the splinter if the skin becomes red, swollen, very painful, or if it bleeds. Get medical help. If the splinter breaks or the victim still feels a piece of splinter below the skin, get medical help.

More on the Subject

Make sure victim is up to date on tetanus immunization (see box opposite). If signs of infection develop — including increased pain, redness, swelling, discharge, swollen lymph nodes, fever, and red streaks spreading from the site toward the heart — get medical help immediately.

Scrapes
(Abrasions)

If skin is scraped against a hard surface, small surface blood vessels will tear and ooze blood. Dirt and bacteria are often ground into the broken skin. If you cannot get a scrape completely clean, or if it looks deep, get medical help.

1. Wash your hands.

2. Scrub the scrape clean with mild soap and a clean washcloth under running water. Try to wash out all the tiny pieces of debris. Use tweezers if necessary (see Splinters, previous section).

3. Apply antibiotic ointment and bandage the injured area.

How to Clean and Bandage a Wound

A wound that is deep or bleeding severely should not be cleaned. Use direct pressure to stop the bleeding (see page 66) and get medical care for the wound.

A wound that is not deep and is not bleeding severely should be cleaned thoroughly to remove contamination before it is dressed and bandaged. This is especially important if medical help will be delayed. The sooner a wound is cleaned, the less likely it is that infection will develop.

All wounds, even minor scrapes and scratches, should be bandaged to protect them from contamination and promote healing.

How to Clean a Wound

First wash your hands thoroughly with soap and running water. Wear sterile gloves if you have them. Then rinse the wound with sterile saline solution or running water. A scrape or shallow scratch should be scrubbed — vigorously, if necessary — with mild soap and a washcloth under running water. Then wipe the wound with first aid antiseptic wipes. Start at the inside of the wound and work toward the edges, using an unused part of the wipe for each stroke.

After the wound has been cleaned, blot it dry with sterile gauze or a clean cloth. If medical help is not needed, apply antibiotic ointment and then bandage the wound. If you cannot get the wound completely clean, bandage the wound and seek medical help as soon as possible.

How to Bandage a Wound

A *dressing* is a sterile covering that is placed directly over a wound. A *bandage* is sometimes needed to hold the dressing in place and support the injured area. Dressings and bandages can be held in place with adhesive tape, masking tape, or improvised cloth ties.

Ideally, you should dress a wound with sterile dressings from your first aid kit. If these are not available, use clean household linen or whatever clean cloth you have on hand. Do not use fluffy cotton on an open wound.

Bandaging Guidelines

- Skin is not sterile. If a dressing slips over the victim's skin while you are trying to position it, discard it and use a fresh dressing. Place the dressing directly on top of the wound; don't slide it into place.
- Use a dressing that is large enough to extend at least 1 inch beyond the edges of the wound.
- If body tissue or organs are exposed, cover the wound with a dressing that will not stick, such as plastic wrap or moistened gauze. Then secure the dressing with adhesive tape until you have medical help.
- If the bandage is over a joint, splint and make a bulky dressing so the joint remains immobilized. If there is no movement of a wound over the joint, there should be improved healing and reduced scarring.
- A bandage should fit snugly but should not cut off circulation or cause the victim discomfort. If the area beyond the wound changes color or begins to tingle or feel cold, or if the wound starts to swell, the bandage is too tight and should be loosened.

Bandaging Techniques

Which bandaging technique you choose depends upon the size and location of the wound, your first aid skills, and the materials you have on hand. There are many advanced bandaging techniques, but the basic principles of bandaging are always the same.

Applying a Basic Dressing/Bandage

If the wound is too big for an adhesive strip (for example, Band-Aid adhesive bandage), cover it with sterile gauze or clean cloth (Figure 87a). Secure the dressing with adhesive tape or, if the wound is on a limb, with a roller bandage or long strip of clean cloth (Figure 87b). Check to be sure the bandage is not too tight (Figure 87c).

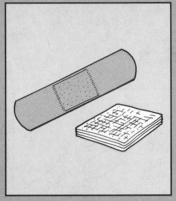
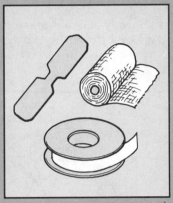
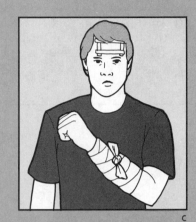

a   b   c

Figure 87 a, b, c
Dressings and bandages

Applying a Roller Bandage

A roller bandage can be used to secure a dressing on a limb (or, if necessary, on the torso). The easiest method is simply to wrap the roller bandage around the limb with spiral turns (Figure 88a). Do not wrap a roller bandage over and over the same place. If more support or pressure is needed, wrap the roller bandage around the limb with crisscross ("figure eight") turns (Figure 88b). Turn under the end of the bandage and secure it with a safety pin, adhesive tape, or clips. If necessary, you can split the end of the roller bandage and use the 2 strips to tie a knot over the wound (Figures 88c and 88d). Check to be sure the bandage is not too tight.

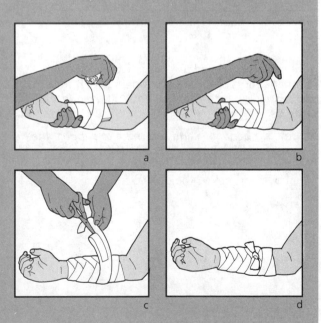

a   b

c   d

Figure 88 a, b, c, d
Applying a roller bandage

(continued)

Applying a Butterfly Bandage

If a wound is gaping slightly but its edges are smooth and even and pull together easily, using a butterfly bandage will speed healing.

You can use a commercial butterfly bandage or make one yourself by trimming a piece of adhesive tape (Figures 89a and 89b). Stick one side of the butterfly bandage to one side of the wound and then gently hold the edges of the wound together before sticking the other side in place.

If the wound is long, you can use two butterfly bandages. On one side of the wound, stick one side of the first bandage; to the other side of the wound, stick one side of the second bandage (Figure 89c). Use the free ends of the bandages to gently pull the wound together before sticking them in place (Figure 89d). Then dress and bandage over the butterfly bandages.

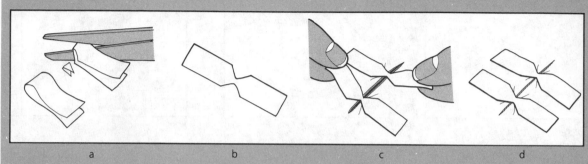

a   b   c   d

Figure 89 a, b, c, d
Making and applying a butterfly bandage

Bandaging an Embedded Object

If an object is embedded in the wound, the bandage must cover the wound and keep the embedded object from moving. You have several options:

- *Roll up bandages and use them to support the embedded object on either side* (Figure 90). Wrap tape firmly around the bandages both above and below the object.

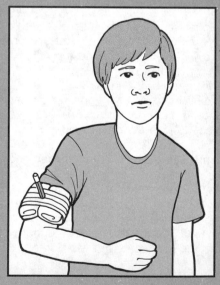

Figure 90
Supporting an embedded object with rolled-up bandages

- *Use a ring bandage to surround the embedded object.* Lightly drape a sterile dressing around the wound and the embedded object (Figures 91a and 91b). Then use a roller bandage or long strip of clean cloth to fashion a ring bandage. The ring should be wide enough to surround the embedded object and high enough to prevent pressure on it (Figure 91c). Secure the ring bandage with another roller bandage (Figure 91d).

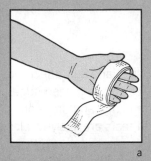 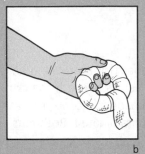 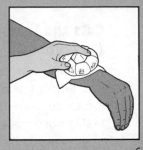 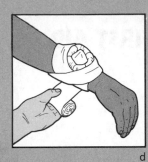

a　　　　　　　　b　　　　　　　　c　　　　　　　　d

Figure 91 a, b, c, d
Supporting an embedded object with a ring bandage

- *Use a paper or Styrofoam cup to cover the embedded object* (Figure 92). Lightly cover the wound with a sterile dressing. Poke a hole in the bottom of the cup and gently place it over the protruding object. Tape the cup in place.

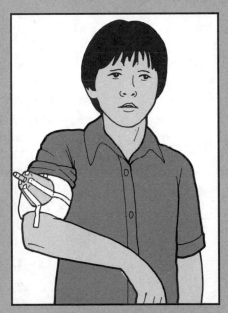

Figure 92
Covering an embedded object with a cup

Make sure the victim is up to date on tetanus immunization. (See box on page 188.) If signs of infection develop — including increased pain, redness, swelling, discharge, swollen lymph nodes, fever, and red streaks spreading from the site toward the heart — get medical help immediately.

FIRST AID

Cuts and Tears
(Lacerations)

Cuts have clean edges (for example, a knife slice) and can affect muscles, tendons, and nerves beneath the skin. Tears have jagged edges, can cause more damage to deeper tissues than cuts, and are more likely to become contaminated. Both cuts and tears are likely to bleed.

- If the victim is seriously injured, call EMS.
- If the victim was bitten by an animal, you will need to determine whether or not it was rabid (see page 58).
- If the wound is deep or bleeding severely, give first aid for bleeding (see **Bleeding** on page 62) and get medical help for care of the wound.
- If the wound is not bleeding severely, give first aid for wounds and get medical help as needed.

DO NOT try to clean a major wound. This can cause heavier bleeding.

DO NOT try to clean a major wound after bleeding has been controlled.

DO NOT assume that a minor wound is clean because you can't see anything inside. Wash it anyway.

DO NOT probe or pull debris from a wound.

DO NOT push body parts back in. Cover them with sterile material (or the cleanest you have) and call EMS.

DO NOT breathe on a wound or dressing.

1. Wash your hands. Wear sterile gloves if you have them.

2. Wash the wound with mild soap and running water.

3. Control bleeding with direct pressure and elevate the injured part above the heart. (See page 66.) *Do not* remove a dressing if it becomes soaked with blood. Instead, add a new dressing on top.

4. If the edges of the wound can be brought together, bandage the wound with a butterfly bandage. (See page 192.) If the wound is ragged, clean and bandage it and get medical help for further care.

More on the Subject

Make sure the victim is up to date on tetanus immunization. (See box on page 188.) If signs of infection develop — including increased pain, redness, swelling, discharge, swollen lymph nodes, fever, and red streaks spreading from the site toward the heart — get medical help immediately.

Puncture Wounds

FIRST AID

A puncture wound is a small but deep hole produced by a pin, nail, fang, bullet, or other penetrating object. It's hard to tell how deep a puncture wound may be. Puncture wounds usually do not cause heavy external bleeding, but they cause internal injury and are at high risk for tetanus infection. (See Tetanus on page 188).

If the victim has an object embedded in a wound, give first aid for Wounds with an Embedded Object (page 196).

- If the victim is seriously injured, call EMS.
- If the victim was bitten by an animal, you will need to determine whether or not it was rabid (see page 58).
- If the wound seems deep or is bleeding severely, give first aid for bleeding (see **Bleeding** on page 62) and get medical help for care of the wound.
- If the wound is not bleeding severely, give first aid for puncture wounds and get medical attention.

DO NOT try to clean a major wound. This can cause heavier bleeding.

DO NOT assume that a minor wound is clean because you can't see anything inside. Wash it anyway.

DO NOT probe or pull debris from a wound.

DO NOT push body parts back in.

DO NOT breathe on a wound or dressing.

1. Wash your hands. Wear sterile gloves if you have them.

2. Rinse the puncture wound thoroughly with a forceful stream of soapy water.

3. Apply antiseptic solution.

4. Bandage the hole with a sterile gauze pad until you have medical help. *Do not* tape the hole closed, and *do not* apply antibiotic ointment. Sealing off the wound can increase the likelihood of infection.

More on the Subject

Make sure the victim is up to date on tetanus immunization. (See box on page 188.) If signs of infection develop — including increased pain, redness, swelling, discharge, swollen lymph nodes, fever, and red streaks spreading from the site toward the heart — get medical help immediately.

FIRST AID

Wounds with an Embedded Object

Any movement of an object that is embedded in a wound may cause further bleeding, damage, and pain. *Do not* move an object that is embedded in a wound. Give first aid and get medical help immediately. If the victim is impaled on a fixed object, prevent him or her from moving until medical help is obtained.

- If the victim is seriously wounded or is impaled on a fixed object, call EMS.

DO NOT pull an embedded object out of a wound.
DO NOT try to clean the wound.
DO NOT breathe on the wound.

1. Leave the object in place.

2. Carefully cut away clothes, if necessary. Any puncture wound that drives through clothes needs medical help.

3. If the object must be cut in order to move the victim, stabilize it and trim it a few inches from the skin.

4. Wash your hands. Wear sterile gloves if you have them.

5. Control bleeding if necessary (see **Bleeding** on page 62), applying indirect pressure to the area around the wound. Do not disturb the embedded object.

6. Immobilize the embedded object with rolled up bandages, a ring bandage, or a paper cup or cone until you have medical help. (See How to Clean and Bandage a Wound on page 190.)

More on the Subject

Make sure the victim is up to date on tetanus immunization. (See box on page 188.) If signs of infection develop — including increased pain, redness, swelling, discharge, swollen lymph nodes, fever, and red streaks spreading from the site toward the heart — get medical help immediately.

Fishhook Removal

If the barb of the fishhook has not entered the skin, pull the tip of the hook out in the same direction it went in. If the barb is embedded under the skin, the first technique to try is the Fish Line Method (following). If this fails and medical help is not available, you will need to use the Wire Cutter Method. (See page 198.)

DO NOT attempt to remove a fishhook if it is embedded near the eye or near an artery.

Fish Line Method

1. Cut a piece of fish line or string approximately 8 inches long.

2. Loop the string around the curved end of the embedded fishhook.

3. Press down on the free (straight) end of the fishhook and at the same time pull on the string (Figure 93a). (If the hook is embedded in a body curve, press down on the middle of the back of the fishhook.) (Figure 93b)

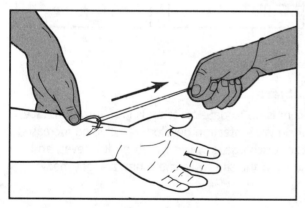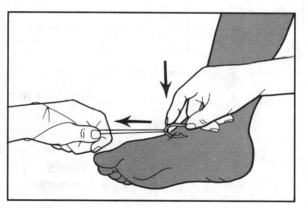

Figure 93 a, b
Removing a fishhook, fish line method

a   b

4. Wash the cut with mild soap and running water and apply an adhesive bandage.

5. Call the victim's physician for advice.

Wire Cutter Method

1. Wash your hands.

2. Push the fishhook through the skin until the barb exits (Figures 94a and 94b).

3. Cut off the barb (Figure 94c). Then pull the rest of the fishhook back out through the entry wound (Figure 94d).

4. Wash the entry and exit wounds vigorously with mild soap and running water.

5. Bandage the wound with a sterile gauze dressing until you have medical help. *Do not* tape the punctures closed or apply antibiotic ointment, since sealing off the wound can increase the likelihood of infection.

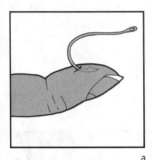 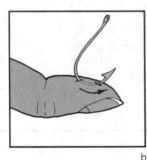 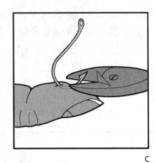 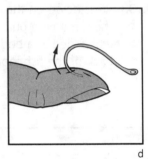

Figure 94 a, b, c, d
Removing a fishhook, wire cutter method

More on the Subject

Make sure the victim is up to date on tetanus immunization. (See box on page 188.) If signs of infection develop — including increased pain, redness, swelling, discharge, swollen lymph nodes, fever, and red streaks spreading from the site toward the heart — get medical help immediately.

FIRST AID

Zipper Injuries

If the skin gets caught in a zipper, *do not* try to pull the skin free. Instead, pop the zipper open by carefully inserting a scissor or other sharp object between the teeth, as far as possible from the skin, taking care not to jab the skin. If you cannot free the skin, get medical help as soon as possible, since trapped skin will start to swell.

CHOKING: ADULT OR CHILD
(Over 1 Year of Age)

1. Ask If Person Is Choking
- If person can't answer, call EMS. Go to Step 2.
- If person is coughing forcefully and can breathe, do not interfere. Stand by.

2. Position Your Hands
- Wrap your arms around person's waist.
- Make a fist. Place thumb side of fist in middle of person's abdomen (above navel and well below lower tip of breastbone) (Fig. 1 inset).

3. Give Abdominal Thrusts
- Grasp fist with other hand.
- Press fist with quick, upward thrusts into abdomen (Fig. 1). Continue until person either starts breathing or loses consciousness.

IF PERSON IS UNCONSCIOUS

4. Call EMS if Someone Hasn't Already

5. Place Person on Back
- Clear mouth if necessary.
- Check for breathing.
  If no breathing . . .

6. Begin Rescue Breathing
- Tilt head back and lift chin (Fig. 2).
- Pinch nose shut.
- Seal your lips tightly around mouth (Fig. 3).
- Give 2 full breaths for 1 to 1½ seconds each.
  If breaths won't go in . . .

OVER

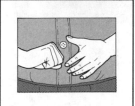

Figure 1

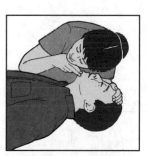

Figure 2

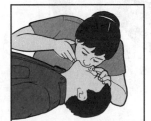

Figure 3

7. Retilt Head and Try Again

- Tilt head farther back.
- Pinch nose shut, seal your lips, and try again to give 2 breaths. *If breaths still won't go in . . .*

8. Give Abdominal Thrusts

- Straddle person's thighs.
- Place heel of hand in middle of abdomen, just above navel and well below lower tip of breastbone.
- Place other hand on top and point fingers toward person's head (Fig. 4).
- Give 6 to 10 quick thrusts inward and upward.

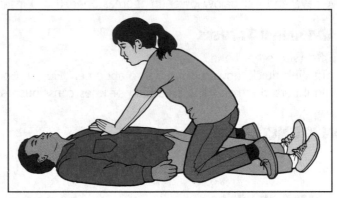

Figure 4

9. Do Finger Sweep

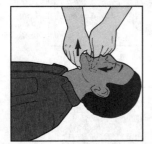

Figure 5

- Grasp tongue and lower jaw. Lift jaw.
- Slide finger down inside cheek to base of tongue (Fig. 5). Sweep object out.
  If person is still not breathing . . .

10. Go Back to Step 6

- Repeat sequence until person begins to cough or breathe.

CHOKING: INFANT
(Newborn to 1 Year of Age)

American Red Cross

1. Is Baby Choking?

- If baby can't cough, breathe, or cry, or is coughing weakly, call EMS. Go to Step 2.
- If baby is coughing forcefully and can breathe, do not interfere. Stand by.

2. Turn Baby Facedown

- Hold baby's jaw and support head as you turn baby facedown.
- Rest your forearm on your thigh.

3. Give 4 Back Blows

- Use the heel of your hand.
- Give 4 blows forcefully between shoulder blades (Fig. 1).

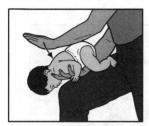

Figure 1

4. Turn Baby onto Back

- Support head.
- Rest baby's back on your thigh.

5. Give 4 Chest Thrusts

- Place index and middle fingers on baby's breastbone, just below nipples (Fig. 2).
- Give 4 quick thrusts down ½ to 1 inch.

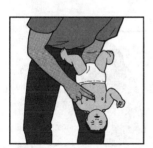

Figure 2

6. Go Back to Step 2

- Repeat sequence until baby coughs up object or starts to cough, cry, or breathe.

IF BABY IS UNCONSCIOUS

7. Call EMS if Someone Hasn't Already

OVER

8. Place Baby on Back

■ Move baby as a unit. Place on firm surface.

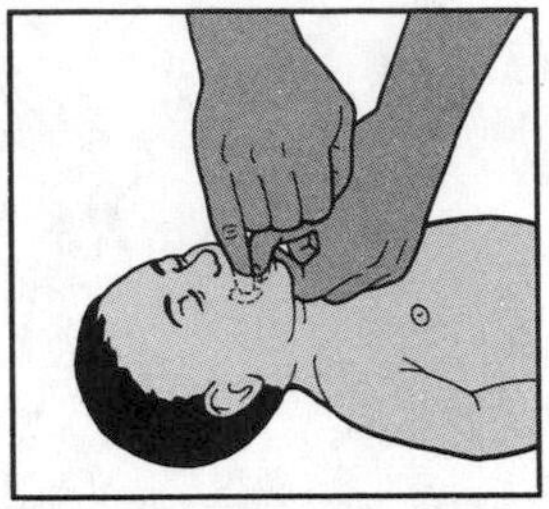

9. Look into Baby's Mouth

■ Grasp tongue and lower jaw. Look for object in mouth.
■ Sweep any object out with your little finger (Figure 3).

10. Begin Rescue Breathing

■ Look. listen, and feel for breathing.
If no breathing . . .
■ Gently tilt head back and lift chin (Fig. 4).
■ Seal your lips tightly around nose and mouth (Fig. 5).
■ Give 2 slow breaths for 1 to 1½ seconds each.
If breaths will not go in . . .

11. Retilt Head and Try Again

■ Tilt head farther back.
■ Seal your lips and try again to give 2 breaths.
If breaths still won't go in, repeat Steps 2 through 6 until airway is cleared or help arrives.

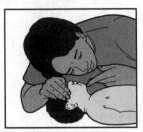

Figure 3

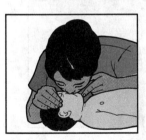

Figure 4

Figure 5

CPR: ADULT

1. Check for Consciousness

- Tap or gently shake person.
- Shout, "Are you OK?"

2. Shout, "Help!"

3. Roll Person onto Back

- Move person as a unit. Support head and neck. Place on firm surface.

4. Open Airway and Check Breathing

- Tilt head back. Lift chin (Fig. 1).
- Look, listen, and feel for breathing for 5 seconds.
  If no breathing . . .

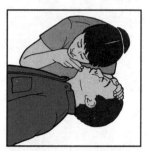

Figure 1

5. Give 2 Full Breaths

- Pinch nose shut.
- Seal your lips tightly around mouth (Fig. 2).
- Give 2 full breaths for 1 to 1½ seconds each.

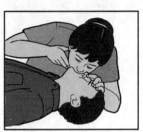

Figure 2

6. Check Pulse

- Feel for pulse at side of neck for 5 to 10 seconds (Fig. 3).
  If no pulse . . .

7. Phone EMS for Help

- Send someone to call.

OVER

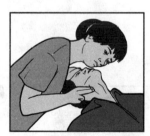

Figure 3

EMERGENCY ACTION GUIDE: CPR

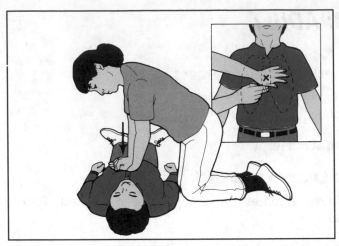

Figure 4

8. Position Your Hands

- Find notch at lower end of breastbone with middle finger.
- Place heel of other hand on breastbone, 2 finger-widths above notch (Fig. 4 inset).
- Remove fingers from notch and place heel of this hand over heel of other hand.
- Keep fingers off chest.

9. Give 15 Compressions

- Lean with shoulders over your hands. Lock your arms (Fig. 4).
- Depress breastbone 1½ to 2 inches.
- Give 15 compressions in 10 seconds.

10. Give 2 Full Breaths

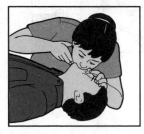

Figure 5

- Tilt head back. Lift chin.
- Pinch nose shut (Fig. 5).
- Give 2 full breaths for 1 to 1½ seconds each.
- Check pulse.
  If no pulse . . .

11. Repeat Cycles of 2 Breaths and 15 Compressions for 4 Cycles

- Continue until person revives or help arrives.

CPR: CHILD
(Age 1 to 8)

1. Check for Consciousness

- Tap or gently shake child.
- Shout, "Are you OK?"

2. Shout, "Help!"

3. Roll Child onto Back

- Move child as a unit. Support head and neck. Place on firm surface.

4. Open Airway and Check Breathing

- Tilt head back. Lift chin (Fig. 1).
- Look, listen, and feel for breathing for 3 to 5 seconds.
  If no breathing . . .

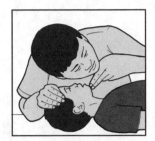

Figure 1

5. Give 2 Slow Breaths

- Pinch nose shut.
- Seal your lips tightly around mouth (Fig. 2).
- Give 2 slow breaths for 1 to 1½ seconds each.

6. Check Pulse

- Use one hand to keep head tilted.
- Feel for pulse at side of neck for 5 to 10 seconds (Fig. 3).
  If no pulse . . .

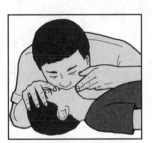

Figure 2

7. Phone EMS for Help

- Send someone to call.

OVER

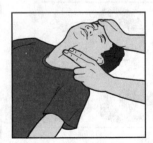

Figure 3

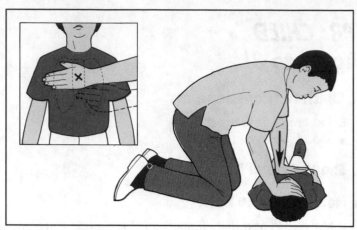

Figure 4

8. Position Your Hands

- Keep head tilted with one hand.
- Find notch at lower end of breastbone with middle finger. Place heel of same hand on breastbone, 2 finger-widths above notch (Fig. 4 inset).
- Keep fingers off chest.

9. Give 5 Compressions

- Lean with shoulder over hand. Lock arm straight (Fig. 4).
- Depress breastbone 1 to 1½ inches.
- Give 5 compressions in about 4 seconds.

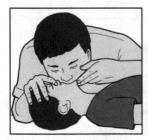

Figure 5

10. Give 1 Slow Breath

- Tilt head back. Lift chin.
- Pinch nose shut.
- Give 1 slow breath for 1 to 1½ seconds (Fig. 5).
- Check pulse.
  If no pulse . . .

11. Repeat Cycles of 1 Breath and 5 Compressions for 10 Cycles.

- Continue until child revives or help arrives.

CPR: INFANT
(Birth to Age 1)

American
Red Cross

1. Check for Consciousness
- Tap or gently shake baby's shoulder.

2. Shout, "Help!"

3. Roll Baby onto Back
- Move baby as a unit. Support head and neck. Place on firm surface.

4. Open Airway and Check Breathing
- Gently tilt head back. Lift chin (Fig. 1).
- Look, listen, and feel for breathing for 3 to 5 seconds. *If no breathing . . .*

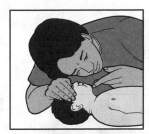
Figure 1

5. Give 2 Slow Breaths
- Seal your lips tightly around nose and mouth (Fig. 2).
- Give 2 slow breaths for 1 to 1½ seconds each.

6. Check Pulse
- Use one hand to keep head tilted.
- Feel for pulse in upper arm for 5 to 10 seconds (Fig. 3). Put your ear close to chest and listen for heartbeat. *If no pulse or heartbeat . . .*

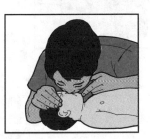
Figure 2

7. Phone EMS for Help
- Send someone to call.

OVER

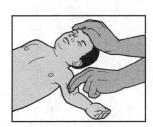
Figure 3

EMERGENCY ACTION GUIDE: CPR

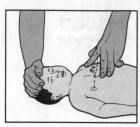

Figure 4

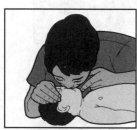

Figure 5

8. Position Your Hands

- Keep head tilted with one hand.
- Place index finger on breastbone, just below nipple level.
- Place next 2 fingers next to index finger, farther down breastbone. Lift index finger (Fig. 4). Use 2 middle fingers for next step.

9. Give 5 Compressions

- Bend your elbow.
- Use 2 fingers to depress breastbone ½ to 1 inch. Push straight down.
- Give 5 compressions in about 3 seconds.

10. Give 1 Slow Breath

- Seal your lips tightly around nose and mouth and give 1 breath (Fig. 5).
- Check pulse.
  If no pulse . . .

11. Repeat Cycles of 1 Breath and 5 Compressions for 10 Cycles

- Continue until baby revives or help arrives.

EXTERNAL BLEEDING

1. Call EMS if Bleeding Is Severe

2. Wash Your Hands

- Wash hands. Put on sterile gloves if you have them.
- Remove loose debris from wound.

3. Apply Direct Pressure

- Put a barrier — layers of sterile dressings, clean cloth, or plastic wrap — between you and wound.
- Press dressing firmly (Fig. 1).
- Don't remove dressing. Put new dressings over soaked dressings. Keep pressing.

4. Elevate

- If no broken bone, raise wound above heart level.
  If person is still bleeding after 15 minutes . . .

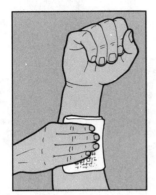

Figure 1

5. Apply Pressure Point Bleeding Control

- Use only when necessary, on arm or leg.
- Find pressure point (feel for pulse) and press artery against the bone (Fig. 2).
- Continue direct pressure and elevation.

6. Prevent Shock

- Lay victim flat. Raise feet. Cover with blanket.

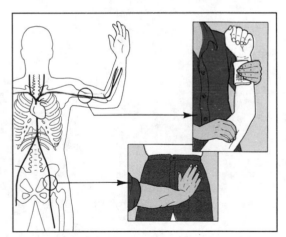

Figure 2

Local emergency (EMS) telephone number_____

When you call EMS, be ready to provide the following information:

- Your name
- Type of emergency
- Location of emergency
- Location of emergency (street address, apartment number, nearby landmarks, major intersections)
- Telephone number you are calling from
- How many are injured

DON'T HANG UP UNTIL THE DISPATCHER TELLS YOU TO!

Personal and Family Safety

In the first two parts of this book, you learned how to cope with the emergencies that inevitably enter our lives. In this part, you'll see many strategies for preventing those emergencies from occurring in the first place.

When it comes to personal health, most of us have become converts to the doctrine of prevention. We try to exercise and avoid unhealthful foods in order to stave off heart disease. We're quitting the cigarette habit in record numbers because we want to avoid the serious health consequences of smoking.

This is a wonderful trend, but avoiding illness is only part of the prevention picture. To lead longer and healthier lives, we must prevent not only illness, but injuries.

If you think about it, most accidents are simply injuries that weren't avoided. We can't stop roads from being slippery, or other drivers from being careless — but we can minimize our risk of being injured by wearing seat belts. We can't stop children from being curious — we wouldn't even want to — but we can put safety latches on cabinet doors and put medicines out of their reach. And while we can't control the forces of nature, there's much we can do to protect ourselves and our families from the devastation of natural disasters.

In the chapters ahead, you'll learn how to make your home a safer place by recognizing potential hazards and doing a room-by-room safety inspection. You'll find out ways to prevent household fires and to prepare for and survive natural disasters. And whether your physical fitness regime takes you to the hiking trail, the tennis court, the swimming pool, or just your own backyard, you'll see that there are many steps you can take to ensure that your enjoyment of a healthy lifestyle does not put you at risk for injury.

If you read this section and put its advice to use, you may even find that you have few occasions to use the first aid advice in the rest of the book. You can prevent most injuries, and you don't have to restrict your activities to do it.

About the Teddy Bear

If children are part of your life, look for the teddy bear in the margin on the pages ahead. It marks sections of the book that provide special safety measures you should take for children.

Household Safety

Chapter

5

More injuries occur in the home than anywhere else, and each year more children die in household injuries than from all childhood diseases combined. The saddest thing about these statistics is that most household accidents are completely preventable.

In this chapter, you'll find a wide array of precautions you can take to make your home a safer place for you and your family. With every safety precaution you take, you reduce the risk of someone becoming injured in your home.

Consider doing a safety inventory of your home. After you've read this section, walk from room to room. Look for danger zones, unsafe practices, harmful objects or substances, and items that might be used in a harmful way. Correct what you can right away, and make a list of other hazards to fix as soon as possible. Pay special attention to the kitchen, bathroom, living room, and family room — these are the areas of greatest activity in the home, and the sites of most injuries.

The very young and the very old are especially at risk for household injuries, so be particularly careful when young children or older people are visiting or living in your home. When you and your family are away from home, try to apply the following household safety precautions to your temporary setting. It will make your stay away from home that much more relaxing and enjoyable.

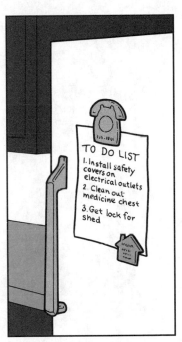

Do a safety inventory of your home.

Using Electricity Safely

Electricity allows us to enjoy many of the conveniences of modern life, but it is also dangerous. Used incorrectly, it can start a house fire or cause serious electrical injuries. Each year in the United States, nearly 1,000 people are killed and thousands more injured as a result of electrical

215

accidents. Your household electrical current is strong enough to kill you outright if you come into contact with it. By familiarizing yourself with the following safety guidelines, you can minimize the risk of any electrical mishap occurring in your home.

- Always position appliances (including televisions, computers, stereos, and heaters) so they have plenty of air space around and under them to prevent overheating. Read and save appliance precautions and instructions.
- Get into the habit of unplugging appliances when they're not in use. During a power failure, unplug all appliances except one (so you can tell when power is restored).
- Unplug appliances during thunderstorms. Electrical appliances can conduct lightning.
- Unplug appliances by grasping the plug, not by yanking on the cord.
- If a plug becomes wet, dry it thoroughly before plugging it back in or using the appliance.
- If an appliance gets wet or is not working correctly, have it serviced.
- Whenever you use an electrical appliance, make sure your hands are dry and that you are not standing in water. Do not let electrical cords run through water.
- Ground any appliance or equipment that requires it.
- Check for visible wear or signs of damage before using any electrical appliance. If the cord is frayed, split, cut, damaged, or hot, the appliance is not safe to use.
- Check your electric blanket and holiday lights each year before using them. Don't leave the lights on overnight.
- Turn the light off before changing a light bulb. Don't use a higher watt bulb than the fixture or lampshade can handle safely.
- Never cover a lampshade with cloth or paper.
- Don't run electrical cords under the rug, where they can become worn or overheated. Position them along the baseboards or walls and behind furniture.
- Don't use an extension cord for a major or heat-producing appliance.
- Don't overload any one extension cord or electrical outlet.
- If you are buying an extension cord, choose one that is rated by the Underwriters Laboratory (UL) and can carry the amount of current you need.

- Make sure outdoor electrical outlets are properly covered.
- If a fuse blows, find out why. A fuse that blows repeatedly or a circuit breaker that trips repeatedly may be a sign of a problem. Short circuits can cause fires. Replace a blown fuse only with a fuse of the same size.

Keeping Children Safe around Electricity

Protect your child from serious electrical injury by taking the following additional precautions:

- Position a child's highchair, playpen, or crib away from electrical outlets, and make sure no wires are within reach.
- Keep all electrical appliances and devices far beyond the reach and climbing range of children.
- Cover all electrical outlets with safety covers. A wide variety of effective outlet covers is now available.
- Buy extension cords that have covers over their outlets — the end of a plugged-in extension cord is "live." They should also have covers over both plugged and unplugged outlets. Keep extension cords out of the reach of children.

How to Poison-Proof Your Home

We all use chemicals every day — from detergents and disinfectants to paints and polishes. Used, stored, and disposed of properly, these household products help keep our homes clean and attractive. But many of the ingredients that make household products effective also make them potentially dangerous, especially if they are used incorrectly or get into the hands of children. By following the guidelines in this section, you can help prevent poisoning and other accidents involving household chemicals from occurring in your home.

Recognizing Poisonous Substances

Poisoning can occur in four ways: through ingestion (swallowing), inhalation (breathing), skin contact, or injection. Your first step in poison-proofing your home is to go through the household products you have on hand and to familiarize yourself with the ways in which they can be harmful. Some are dangerous in small amounts; others are hazardous in quantity. Some are poisonous if swallowed; others give off harmful vapors. Starting with your kitchen, go through your home room by room, checking shelves and reading labels (some may surprise you!). If you're in doubt about a product, call your local Poison Control Center.

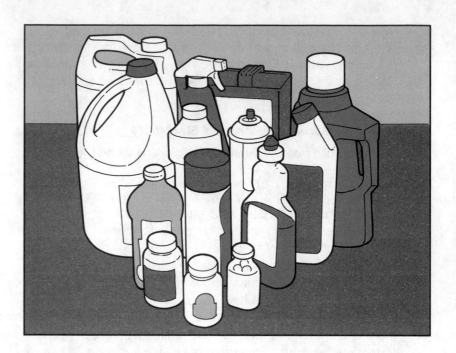

Be aware of the potentially toxic substances in your home.

Potentially Toxic Substances

Here is a partial list of some of the potentially poisonous products commonly found in the home:

Acetaminophen (pain reliever)
Air freshener
Alcohol (rubbing) and alcoholic
 beverages
Ammonia
Antifreeze
Aspirin
Bleach
Boric acid
Cleaning fluids
Cleansers
Cosmetics
Deodorants, deodorizers
Dishwasher detergents
Disinfectants
Drain cleaners
Fabric softener
Felt-tip marker pens
Fertilizer
Flaking paint

Floor polish
Furniture polish
Gasoline
Hair dyes
Herbal or home remedies
Insecticides
Insulation
Kerosene
Laundry detergent
Lighter fluid
Lime
Linseed oil
Lye
Medications of any kind
Metal cleaner or polish
Mothballs
Nail polish, nail polish
 remover
Oven cleaner
Paint

Paint remover
Perfume, cologne,
  aftershave
Pesticides
Plants
Polishes and waxes
Rat poison
Roach killer
Soaps and shampoos

Solvents
Suntan lotions
Tobacco products
Toilet bowl cleaners
Turpentine
Varnishes
Vitamins
Weed killers
Window cleaners

Using and Storing Household Products Safely

Never be casual about potentially dangerous household products, and never use them in a hurry. Respect them. Read labels, follow instructions exactly, and store these substances carefully.

Some guidelines:

- Buy potentially poisonous substances in safety containers, and buy only as much as you need.
- Store all household products in their original containers. Don't transfer household products into unsuitable or unmarked containers. *Never* store household products in food or drink containers.
- Do not use potentially toxic substances in the kitchen or around food.
- Store all household products safely immediately after use.
- Never mix household products. For example, many cleaners contain either ammonia or bleach, which can let off a toxic gas when combined.
- Use products that give off fumes — including ammonia, bleach, petroleum products, and paints — only in well-ventilated areas.
- Make sure you have adequate ventilation around any fuel-burning appliances and be sure they are working correctly. When they are operating, these appliances release poisonous carbon monoxide gas that needs to be dispersed into the air.
- Store all household products out of the reach of children, preferably in a locked cabinet.
- Never store household products, particularly aerosols, near a source of heat or flame such as a furnace or hot water heater.

Using Medicines Safely

Medicines are wonderful and at times miraculous tools in preventing and curing disease, but only when taken as directed. Both prescription and over-the-counter medications can be extremely dangerous if they are used incorrectly. In fact, the most common poisoning emergencies involve medicines. With that in mind:

- Buy medications with childproof caps.
- Never take or administer any medication that has no label, that is out of date, that has begun to crumble, or that has changed color, odor, or consistency.
- Don't take or administer any medication in the dark or in the presence of children.
- Don't give a prescription medication to anyone other than the person for whom it was prescribed.
- The bathroom cabinet isn't the best place to store medicines. A locked box kept in a dry, cool place out of the reach of children is best.
- Clean out your medicine chest regularly. Dispose of old medicines by flushing them down the toilet.
- Make sure each prescription medication is clearly labeled by the pharmacist with instructions for its use and its expiration date.
- Do not reuse old medicine bottles.
- Always be sure you understand what a drug is, how it works, when and how to take it, and what the potential side effects are.
- Mixing medications and alcohol can be deadly. Don't do it except under the advice of a physician or pharmacist.

Keeping Children Safe from Poisoning

Nearly 75 percent of all poisonings in children are due to household agents. Products not kept out of the sight and reach of children can cause an emergency.

Children under five are especially at risk for poisoning accidents. They are curious, they are not concerned about what's poisonous and what isn't, and they will eat or drink almost anything. Even the best-behaved child is not safe if a poisonous substance is within his or her reach.

Here are some additional guidelines to keep in mind if children are in your home:

- Buy poisonous substances and medicines in child-resistant containers, but don't rely solely upon them. Store *any* dangerous product in a locked cabinet out of the reach of children.
- Be careful where you leave a dangerous substance. If you're interrupted in the middle of a project, put away any hazardous products with which you are working. Never leave medicines on your bedside table or in your purse.

- Never tell children that medicine tastes like candy.
- Never leave a child alone with any medication, even if it's in a child-resistant container.
- Keep aerosol spray cans out of reach. Both the propellant and the product may be poisonous.
- Have houseguests lock up their medications during their stay.
- Teach your child that plants are to look at, not to eat. (See page 259 for more on poisonous plants.)

Preventing Food Poisoning

If you eat food that contains certain viruses, bacteria, or their toxic by-products, you will get sick. The general term for this is "food poisoning." You can take steps to prevent food poisoning by buying, preparing, and storing foods correctly.

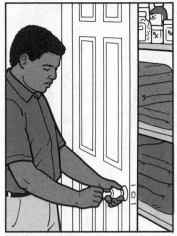

Store dangerous products in a locked cabinet.

- Carefully examine all food containers. Discard a can if the seams are dented, rusted, swollen, or leaking. Don't eat anything from a glass jar that is cracked, chipped, or has a swollen lid. Don't eat any food packed in paper that has stains, cuts, or leaks. Never eat a product that may have been tampered with.
- Keep food refrigerated below 40° Fahrenheit.
- Check expiration dates on packaged foods. "Sell by . . ." allows sufficient time after purchase for home use under proper storage conditions. "Best if used by . . ." is the manufacturer's determination of how long the product will still be good. "Expiration date" is the last day an item should be used.
- Always wash your hands thoroughly before and after preparing food, especially if you are handling raw meat, poultry, or fish. To prevent the spread of bacteria, dry your hands with a clean, dry towel (damp dishtowels can be a source of contamination).
- Rinse and dry the tops of canned goods before opening.
- Carefully rinse fruits, vegetables, and raw poultry and fish before preparing or eating them.
- Make sure counter tops, cutting boards, and utensils are clean each time you use them, especially after contact with raw meat, poultry, or fish. Wipe them with a disinfectant cleaner and hot water. Plastic cutting boards are better for use with meat, fish, and poultry since bacteria are less likely to get into cracks.
- Cook meat, seafood, poultry, and eggs thoroughly. Defrost frozen meats completely in the refrigerator, not at room temperature. Be sure the inside cooks through.
- Avoid raw meat, seafood, and eggs.

- Keep hot foods hot (at or above 140° Fahrenheit) and cold foods cold. Never leave food standing, since bacteria thrive in lukewarm food. Serve hot dishes straight from the stove or oven; put leftovers away immediately. (Throw away perishable leftovers left out for more than two hours.)
- Store leftovers from a hot meal in shallow containers. They'll cool through quickly and bacteria will not have a chance to multiply.
- Prepared salads, salad dressings, custards, and pastries all spoil quickly. Refrigerate them immediately after making them, and keep them refrigerated until just before serving.
- Freeze food quickly in airtight containers. Make sure your freezer is working efficiently and that the food freezes within 24 hours. Small packets of food freeze more quickly than large ones.
- When canning food, use reliable instructions and follow them exactly. Don't use shortcuts. Whenever possible, don't use the open-kettle method. Cook foods thoroughly, and don't allow them to cool before bottling them. Use proper jars and lids to create a good seal.
- Bulging cans, even if home canned, should not be opened. If a food smells strange, do not even taste it. If you are in any way suspicious about the taste of prepared food, do not eat it.

Household Safety Precautions

Sometimes the simplest precaution protects you from the greatest harm. In the following pages, you'll find room-by-room descriptions of common-sense measures you can take to make your home a safer place — starting today!

Kitchen

The kitchen is usually one of the busiest areas of the house. It also contains all kinds of dangers — hot grease, boiling liquids, sharp knives, and poisons, to name a few — so the kitchen is clearly not the place to be careless.

General Safety Precautions

- Store cleaners and other household products in locked cabinets away from food products and out of the reach of children.
- Wipe up any spills immediately.

- Turn the handles of pots toward the back of the stove while cooking.
- When buying a stove, choose one with knobs at the back.
- Never hang anything flammable above gas burners, and don't wear clothes with loose sleeves while cooking.
- Keep cabinet doors closed, since their sharp corners near eye level can be dangerous.
- Keep a supply of sturdy hot pads within easy reach.
- If you're called away while ironing, turn off the iron and place it out of the reach of children.

Child-proofing Your Kitchen

- Never leave children alone in the kitchen.
- Make sure anything sharp, poisonous, heavy, or breakable is out of the reach of children. Store dangerous foods (such as nuts, hard candies, or extracts) on your highest shelves. Don't store tempting foods such as cookies near the stove. Put safety locks on kitchen cabinets and drawers.

- Push small appliances well back on countertops.
- Keep the doors locked on any potential hiding place — broom closet, dishwasher, freezer, washer, dryer — so children cannot accidentally close themselves inside.
- If you have inside doors that lock, be sure you have a key for each one. Another way to keep children out of dangerous areas is to install hook-and-eye latches above the reach of children.
- Store plastic bags out of the reach of children. Tie knots in plastic bags before throwing them away.
- Don't use a tablecloth, since a child can pull it, along with hot food and dishes, onto his or her head. Position things out of reach in the center of the kitchen table. Don't put *hot* liquids such as coffee near the edge of tables, counters, or other surfaces.
- Do not keep medications, including vitamins, on the kitchen table.
- Use the back burners of the stove when cooking. If your stove has knobs on the front edge, cover them with safety covers, or remove them entirely when not in use and keep them in a safe place. You can also buy a stove guard that encircles the top of the stove.

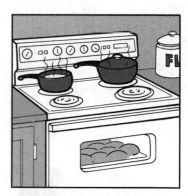

Turn pot handles toward the back of the stove.

- Choose a garbage can that children cannot open, and take extra care when disposing of hazardous substances, broken glass, or cans with sharp edges.
- Put your iron to cool in a safe place out of the reach of children. Never leave it on the ironing board with the cord dangling down.
- Buy unbreakable plates and mugs for children.
- Make sure animal doors are secure or so small that children can't crawl through them.

Living Room/Stairs

Trips and falls are a concern in the living room and on the stairs. Since the injuries associated with falling can be serious, it is a good idea to make it as easy to move around inside your home as possible.

General Safety Precautions

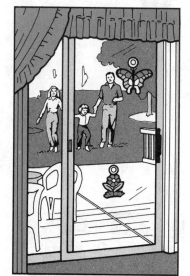

- Put rubber backing under area rugs to keep them from slipping.
- Never allow a fire in a fireplace to burn itself out without anyone watching.
- Make sure there are no electrical cords trailing across the floor or under rugs.
- Put decals at the eye level of both adults and children on glass patio doors.
- Be sure the stairs are well lighted. There should be light switches at both the top and bottom.
- Keep the steps free of clutter.
- If the stairs are carpeted, make sure the carpet is secure and there are no raised edges to trip over.
- Be sure each staircase has a sturdy railing.
- Don't have a glass door at the bottom of the stairs.

Put decals at eye level on glass doors.

Child-proofing Your Living Room/Stairs

- Make sure the fireplace (or woodburning stove, or heater) is well screened. Lock up the matches.
- Position knickknacks and sharp objects out of reach. Don't keep poisonous house plants, and don't leave out dishes of nuts or small candies.
- Lie down on the floor and look for potential hazards, such as nails sticking out of furniture or small objects on the floor.
- Put cords from draperies or blinds out of reach.
- Put guards on sharp furniture corners.
- Install radiator covers to help prevent burns.

- Make sure large objects (bookcases, heavy lamps, etc.) cannot tip over.
- Put mesh (not accordion style) gates at the top and bottom of stairs. Check banister supports to be sure a child's head cannot fit through them. The supports should be less than four inches apart.

Bathroom

Like the kitchen, the bathroom is an area of the house that gets a lot of use and also poses many dangers. Risks in the bathroom include slipping, scalding, poisoning, and electrocution — a frightening list! Fortunately it is easy to avoid these dangers by taking a few commonsense precautions.

General Safety Precautions

- Put nonskid mats inside and nonslip bathmats outside the tub or shower.
- Install handles along the wall of the tub or shower and beside the toilet, particularly if there are older people in the household.
- Position electrical outlets far from the bath. Install ground fault interruptor (GFI) outlets, a special kind of safety outlet that prevents shocks. When possible, use battery-operated appliances in the bathroom.
- Set your hot water heater so the water will not scald (under 120° Fahrenheit).
- Use unbreakable bottles, containers, and cups.
- Wipe up spilled water promptly.
- Ventilate the bathroom while cleaning it.

Child-proofing Your Bathroom

- Never leave children unattended near a bathtub that has water in it.
- If you have separate faucets, run cold water into the tub first, then add hot. This way a child cannot step into a scalding bath.
- The bathroom contains many dangerous items. Lock up medications, razors, cleaning products, and drain cleaner. Put bubble bath, cologne, cosmetics, and other potentially hazardous products on high shelves out of the reach of children.
- Install a safety lock to keep the toilet lid down.
- If you have shower doors, be sure they are made of plastic or tempered glass and covered with safety film. Add decals for good measure.

Bedroom

Falls are common in the bedroom. One reason for this is that you are likely to be walking around your room in the dark. You can reduce your risk of falling by being on the lookout for awkwardly placed furniture and other hazards that might trip you.

General Safety Precautions

- Use a night-light to light your way in the dark, and keep a flashlight in a bedside table in case of a power outage.
- Check for trailing electrical cords that might trip you.
- Make sure bedside lamps are stable, or use wall-mounted lamps.
- *Never* smoke in bed.

Child-proofing a Child's Bedroom

- Do not place furniture that children can climb on in front of a window.
- Choose stable pieces of furniture that will not tip over. Wall-mounted lamps cannot tip over.
- Secure all curtain or blind cords out of children's reach from both floor and crib heights.
- Never use plastic bags or any thin plastic material to cover a mattress.
- Position the crib away from electrical outlets, lamps, and pictures. Do not leave any large objects inside the crib, including pillows. Take toys out of the crib while the baby sleeps.
- Remove any crib gym as soon as your child is able to get up on his or her hands and knees.
- Buy flame-retardant curtains, nightclothes, and bedding.
- Toy chests should have safety lids that cannot lock your child inside or fall on his or her fingers. Air holes are also important should your child ever get inside. Better yet, keep toys on shelves the child can reach.

Storage Areas

Storage areas such as basements, garages, toolsheds, and even hall closets can present hazards to both adults and children, in part because their contents are out of sight — and therefore out of mind.

General Safety Precautions

- Don't let storage areas become so crowded that contents spill out when doors are opened. (If you haven't used it in a year, you probably won't.)
- Use care in storing lawn and garden chemicals, paint supplies, swimming pool chemicals, and other hazardous materials. Make a habit of searching the label for information on storage requirements. Call your sanitation department for information on disposing of hazardous materials. Keep hazardous materials in a locked area.
- If tools are stored on pegboards, be sure that hooks and catches are secure.
- Engage safety devices, such as latches on clipping shears, before storing.
- Hang safety glasses in plain sight near the door so you will remember to use them.

Child-proofing Storage Areas

- Keep storage areas securely locked.
- If tools are stored in an area the child walks through, such as a basement or garage, be sure they cannot drop onto the child. Never permit your child to play alone in such an area.
- If children are helping with chores, retrieve and put away the tools they will need yourself. Inspect any tool you intend to give a child for splinters, sharp edges, and loose parts.
- Locks are available to disable many power tools. Check with a lock shop or hardware store.

Living Safely with Children: An Injury Prevention Plan

Caring for children is tricky. On one hand, you must ensure their safety; but on the other hand, you must allow them to grow and challenge themselves. It's difficult to get the right balance. The following five-point injury prevention plan should help you find a safe middle ground in which your child will flourish.

1) *Never underestimate what a child can do.* A newborn cannot fall off a bed, right? Wrong. A child cannot open a child-resistant container, right? Wrong again! Children learn fast, so play it safe and assume that your child is more mobile and more dexterous than you thought possible.

2) *Recognize what is age-appropriate for each child.* Your household safety precautions need to keep pace with your child. It is important to be ready for the day your child masters a new skill — for example,

climbing out of the crib or opening the front door. It's equally important, however, not to assume your child is capable of handling a situation that is too advanced for him or her.

When choosing toys, keep in mind that the ages designated on the package represent not just intellectual age but also physical age. Adults often think a two-year-old is "advanced" and buy toys labeled for a three- or four-year-old — with small parts that can be put in mouths, ears, or noses.

3) *Create a safe environment.* If you have read the rest of this chapter, you already know how to provide a safe and secure home environment for children. You can do a great deal to keep a child from physical harm by removing dangers from his or her presence.

4) *Supervise children carefully.* There is *no* substitute for adequate supervision, no matter how safe the environment or situation appears to be. Know where your children are and what they are doing at all times.

5) *Teach safety.* Your goal is to help your child learn how to look out for himself or herself. If you explain safety precautions and consistently reinforce safe behavior, eventually your child will be able to make sound decisions about his or her own well-being.

To supplement this plan and the household child-proofing precautions you've just reviewed, here are some age-appropriate safety guidelines for growing children.

Infants (Birth to 1 Year of Age)

Babies progress quickly at this age. Within a year, a helpless newborn becomes an extremely capable little person. Your challenge is always to stay one step ahead.

- Never leave a baby unattended on a bed, table, or other surface the baby could roll off.
- Never leave a baby in a mesh playpen with one side down.
- To reduce the risk of choking accidents, make sure children do not come into contact with small objects such as buttons, watch batteries, popcorn, coins, grapes, or nuts. It is also important to sit with a child as he or she eats. Do not prop bottles, and do not allow a child to crawl or toddle around while eating.
- Don't give infants toys that are heavy or fragile or that have batteries or small parts.
- Supervise babies around furniture and near water.
- Never tie pacifiers (or anything else) around a baby's neck.
- Start teaching your child the meaning of *"Don't touch."* The earliest safety lesson is *"No!"*

Toddlers and Preschoolers (Age 1 to 5)

Young children are mobile and curious, always experimenting with their environment. They have an unreliable grasp of cause and effect, and they are just as likely to forget an important safety measure as to remember it.

- Think ahead to what your child may get into next, and be ready.
- Climbing and squirming are to be expected at this age. Always use safety straps on high chairs and strollers.
- Dangers such as electrical outlets, stovetops, and medicine cabinets are particularly attractive to an inquisitive child. Child-proof and poison-proof your entire home carefully.
- Inspect toys for fragility, small parts, sharp edges, projectiles, and other hazards.
- Choose nontoxic paints, markers, crayons, etc.
- Teach preschoolers the basic principles of fire safety. (See page 238.)
- Teach young children the importance of water safety rules. (See Chapter 9, Water Safety.) Never, *ever* take your eyes from a child near water.

Older Children (Age 5 to 9)

By this age, your child should have a reasonably firm grasp of your household's basic safety rules. He or she is getting more independent and needs to know how to get around safely alone.

- Teach your child to swim.
- Teach your child pedestrian safety (see page 286) and bicycle safety (see page 270).
- Show your child how to use new toys safely.
- Since your child will probably be spending more time alone in his or her room or playroom, make sure you have removed all potential dangers from these areas. If he or she spends time playing alone in the yard, make sure this area is safe as well. (See page 257.)
- It's best not to have guns in a home with children, but if you do have a gun, purchase a trigger lock, keep it in a locked cabinet, and keep ammunition locked up in a separate place.

A Baby-Sitter Checklist

You probably have a list of dos and don'ts to review with your baby-sitters. Here's a safety checklist that should be part of your routine, before you walk out the door. You will find it useful whether you plan to be away for an evening or a week.

- Make sure your Emergency Information Chart (Appendix B) is posted by the phone. Leave a pad and pencil, and write down the number where you can be reached as well as the number of a friend, neighbor, or relative who can help in an emergency. Tell the baby-sitter to get help *first* in an emergency, then call you. Assure the baby-sitter that it is better to overreact than to take unnecessary risks.
- Leave a Consent and Contact Form (Appendix C) and information about your medical insurance coverage in case your child needs to receive medical treatment in your absence. If your child has any allergies or ongoing medical conditions, leave this information as well, since it could affect treatment.
- Tell the baby-sitter about any current health problems your child has and any medication he or she is taking. Make sure the baby-sitter knows how to correctly administer any medications that must be given. Leave written instructions that state where the medicine is kept, when it should be administered, and how much your child should be given. If possible, measure the dosage yourself before you leave. Have the baby-sitter write down what he or she gave your child and when.
- Review basic first aid procedures with the baby-sitter and show him or her where you keep this book and your first aid kit. Post the tear-out Emergency Action Guides. Go over the quickest route to the nearest hospital, just in case.
- Show the baby-sitter around your home. The baby-sitter should know the location of:

Thermostats	Fuse box or circuit breakers
Light switches	Flashlight
Telephone	Keys to inside doors
Danger areas	

- Review fire safety guidelines with the baby-sitter. (See Chapter 6.) Show where you keep your fire extinguisher and how to operate it. Point out any fire exits and the escape routes you have planned. Tell the baby-sitter the outside meeting place your family has agreed upon, and be sure he or she knows how to call the fire department. Make sure that the baby-sitter knows that he or she should get the children out of the house as soon as anyone smells smoke or a fire breaks out.
- Tell your baby-sitter how to keep your home safe from intruders. If you have a security system, the sitter should know how to operate it. Explain how he or she should answer the telephone and the door. If you are expecting any calls, visitors, or deliveries, tell the baby-sitter.
- If the baby-sitter will be giving your child a bath, review safe bathing procedures.
- Give the baby-sitter specific instructions on how to operate household appliances. If any appliances are off limits, say so.
- If you are going to be away for more than a day or an evening, arrange for another person — a neighbor or relative — to check on the baby-sitter.

Fire Prevention, Preparedness, and Survival

According to the National Fire Protection Association, the United States has one of the highest death rates from fire in the world, and fire is the second leading cause of accidental death in the home. Each year there are more than 2 million residential fires, resulting in more than 6,000 deaths. These are appalling statistics, especially when you consider that we can not only prevent fires but also save lives by being prepared.

To begin, let's look at the various preventive measures you can take to minimize the chance you'll ever have to face a fire.

Fire Prevention

A good starting point in your fire prevention campaign is to become familiar with the most common sources of fires within the home. These include:

- Cigarettes and matches
- Cooking equipment
- Kitchen grease
- Home heating equipment
- Flammable items used or stored incorrectly
- Electrical short circuits
- Overheated electrical appliances

(*Note:* Electrical hazards are discussed separately on page 215.)

Cigarettes

Though small, cigarettes, cigars, pipes, matches, and cigarette lighters can generate enough heat to cause a burn or start a serious blaze. Smoking and the improper disposal of smoking materials are the leading causes of fatal home fires in the United States: each year approximately 250,000 house fires are caused by smoking materials, and nearly 2,000 lives are lost as a result.

The following guidelines will help you prevent these tragedies in your home:

- Never smoke in bed!
- Never let ashes, or lit cigarettes, cigars, or pipes, rest on furniture.
- Don't let children play with matches or cigarette lighters. Tell them always to give matches to adults.
- Before emptying the contents of an ashtray, fill the ashtray with water to be sure all the butts are completely extinguished.
- Never empty an ashtray into a trash can that has waste paper in it.
- Designate one metal trash can for all ashes and cigarette and cigar butts. Routine trash can go into plastic waste baskets, but ashtrays should be emptied into a metal trash can.

Kitchen Fires

Most kitchen fires start when cooking food is left unattended. You can prevent most of these fires (and, not incidentally, serious burns) by keeping a close eye on any food that is cooking.

Here are some additional safety measures to keep in mind:

- Have an ABC-type of fire extinguisher handy in your kitchen.
- Pay especially close attention to hot grease, which can self-ignite. Heat oil slowly and watch your cooking temperature. Don't overfill deep fat fryers or skillets.
- Keep flammable items away from the stove, and don't let anything dangle near the heat source while you are cooking (for example, long sleeves, curtains, or even plastic jewelry).
- Keep your heat-producing appliances clean. Old food particles and greasy buildup can ignite.
- Don't let your pressure cooker boil dry.
- Don't put anything on top of your stove except cookware. A pot holder near a hot burner is a fire hazard.
- If you think your gas stove is leaking gas, call the gas company — do not check by lighting a match. If there really is a gas leak, this could cause an explosion.

To keep small kitchen fires from spreading, remember the following guidelines:

- If a fire breaks out in a cooking pan, quickly place the lid over

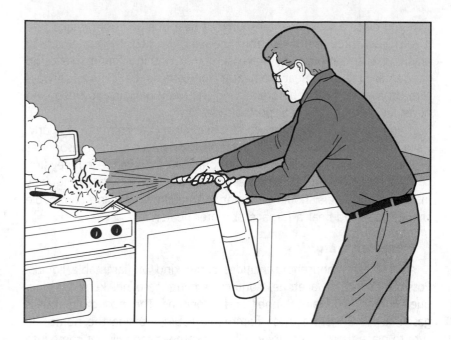

Keep a fire extinguisher in your kitchen.

it, if you can do so safely. This will contain the fire and put it out. *Do not* pour water on a grease fire.

- If something in your oven catches fire, close the oven door to suffocate the flames. Then turn off the oven.
- If something in your microwave is on fire, keep the door closed until it goes out. If you open the door to get at the problem, the air rushing in will feed the fire.

Home Heating

Home heating equipment accidents are a major cause of home fires. Before you buy supplemental home heating equipment — for example, a wood stove, kerosene heater, gas-fired space heater, or portable electric heater — check with your fire department for local fire and building codes. Choose a portable heater that has a wide base and that will turn off automatically if it is tipped over. Buy tested and labeled equipment, and read and follow the manufacturer's instructions. Most manufacturers give a toll-free phone number you can call for assistance. If you have any doubts, don't take chances; call for the correct information.

Use only the fuel recommended by the manufacturer — for example, only wood in a wood stove, only kerosene in a kerosene heater. Never, ever use gasoline in a home heating appliance. Before refilling a heater that runs on liquid fuel, make sure the appliance has cooled down.

If you place a supplemental source of heat in a bedroom, make sure it is at least three feet away from the wall, the bed, the curtains, and anything else combustible. Make sure that nothing flammable could accidentally fall on or near the heater (for example, bedclothes). Always turn off a space heater before leaving the room or going to sleep, and never let children play near portable heaters.

If you have a fireplace or wood stove, clean the chimney regularly. Have your chimney periodically inspected for cracks in the masonry as well as soot buildup. A dirty chimney could cause a sudden chimney fire.

Your home heating system, gas, oil, or electric, should be regularly inspected and filters should be changed frequently. Nothing flammable should be stored near a furnace or water heater.

Flammable Liquids

Almost every household includes some kind of flammable liquids. Possibilities include acetone, contact cement, gasoline, kerosene, lacquer, lighter fluid, paint thinner, and turpentine. The most dangerous is gasoline. Always store these flammable liquids outside the home. Be sure to place them where they will not overheat and will not come into contact with a heat source. Keep in mind that these products produce invisible vapors that can ignite. Even a small spark produced some distance away can cause a sudden blaze. Never use any flammable liquid as an indoor cleaner.

Lightning

With enough volts to light up the night skies, split trees from top to bottom, and ignite fires instantly, lightning is indeed a force to be respected. Make sure your home has lightning rods; these will direct lightning harmlessly into the ground. Lightning tends to strike electrical appliances that are plugged in, so when a severe thunderstorm is approaching, unplug your television and other appliances. (See Lightning on page 248.)

Fire Preparedness

Despite your precautions, you may someday have a fire in your home. If you face this possibility head on, there are very real benefits. The emergency plans you make today may save your family and home tomorrow.

There are three key aspects of fire preparedness: smoke detectors, fire extinguishers, and escape plans.

Choosing Flame-resistant Products

Even a small fire within the home can quickly turn into an inferno if it ignites nearby flammable materials. Any buildup of old rags, boxes, or newspapers is a serious fire hazard. In the kitchen, a fire can rapidly spread to pot holders, dish towels, curtains, or paper goods. Furniture, bedding, curtains, and clothing can all go up in flames.

You can help prevent a fire from spreading by choosing flame-resistant products for your home. Buy upholstered furniture that has a gold tag indicating that the item has been manufactured to comply with the requirements of the Upholstered Furniture Action Council. (Keep in mind that although today's upholstered furniture is less likely to ignite than the furniture of ten years ago, it is *not* fireproof.) When you buy anything labeled flame resistant, follow the manufacturer's cleaning instructions to maintain this feature.

When you choose clothing, be aware that some fibers burn more quickly than others. You should avoid wearing them when cooking or around open flames. Polyester fabrics can cause serious burns because as they burn, the material melts and continues to burn into the skin. Loose, flowing garments catch fire more easily than trim ones. Keep in mind, too, that wearing clothes that can be quickly removed (as opposed to clothes that go over the head or are difficult to take off) can prevent serious burns to the skin.

Smoke Detectors

Smoke detectors are a must in your home. These devices detect the first whiffs of smoke and give you the earliest possible warning by sounding an alarm. If you're asleep — and fires often start while people are sleeping — the alarm will awaken you. Smoke detectors are easy to purchase and install, and they don't cost much, particularly when you consider what they are protecting. In some areas, they are required by law. Check with your fire department to see what your local laws require.

There are three kinds of devices available: heat detectors, flame detectors, and smoke detectors. Smoke detectors are the most suitable for the home. Most are battery powered for easy installation.

Start by putting detectors on each level of your home, as well as in the garage, utility room, and workshop. Read the manufacturer's instructions regarding how and where to install your smoke detector. It is usually a good idea to install a smoke detector at the top of each stairway; since smoke rises, it will probably pass by the alarm. At the top of the base-

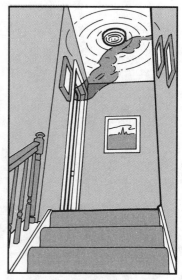

Install a smoke detector on each level of your home.

ment stairs, however, there may be dead air space in front of a closed door, so install a basement alarm lower down. Make sure you can hear your smoke alarms over any other household noise (for example, air conditioning).

If you take good care of your smoke detector, it will take good care of you. Never disconnect it or turn it off. Clean it regularly — dust and grease can build up inside. To remove dust, blow carefully or gently vacuum the interior. Batteries usually last at least six months, but it's important to test them once a month by activating the test button. Keep extra batteries on hand so you can replace dead batteries immediately. When the batteries are dead, the smoke detector will begin to beep or chirp every few seconds or so (the sound is clearly different from an actual alarm). Don't ignore this warning. In fact, you may want to change the batteries regularly. An easy plan is to do it each spring and fall when you reset your clocks.

Fire Extinguishers

A portable fire extinguisher is your best defense against a small home fire. *Do not* throw water on a kitchen fire or electrical fire; this can actually worsen the blaze, particularly if grease is burning. Instead, use a chemical fire extinguisher.

Fire extinguishers are divided into four classes, according to how they should be used:

- Class A is for use on paper, wood, trash, cloth, upholstery, rubber, and other ordinary materials that burn easily.
- Class B is for use on fuel oil, gas, paint, solvents, and other flammable liquids.
- Class C is for use on electrical equipment, fuse boxes, wiring, and appliances.
- Class D is for use on metals.

A combination fire extinguisher is multipurpose. For example, a BC extinguisher is appropriate for kitchen or electrical fires, and an ABC extinguisher is a good choice for an all-purpose home fire extinguisher. Choose carefully, since using the wrong type of fire extinguisher — for example, a Class A extinguisher on a grease fire — can actually make a fire worse.

Fire extinguishers are also rated according to the size of the fire they can put out. The higher the number that precedes the classification (for example, 3BC), the greater the extinguisher's capability. However, fire extinguishers that can cover more area also tend to be heavier. If you can't lift an extinguisher easily, buy a smaller size.

Many fire extinguishers come with a pressure gauge. Check the pressure often, because the extinguisher won't work correctly unless the pressure is up to the proper operating level. If the extinguisher loses pressure it will need to be recharged, repaired, or replaced. Even if you use a pressurized fire extinguisher just briefly, you still need to recharge it afterward.

Purchase only fire extinguishers that have an Underwriters Laboratory (UL) label. Your local fire department can help you with your choice and give you advice on the proper use of fire extinguishers.

Install fire extinguishers in your home near any possible fire hazards. Make sure the extinguishers are easily accessible. It's also a good idea to keep fire extinguishers in your car, boat, or motor home. Be sure you know how to operate them! Use a back-and-forth motion at the base of the flame. Fire extinguishers are made to put out small fires. If a fire is not quickly extinguished, call your fire department immediately.

Home Escape Plans

Few things are more terrifying than fire. If you and your family have practiced fire drills in advance, you'll be able to act quickly and make the correct decisions during a real fire, thereby saving precious seconds and even lives.

Start your emergency planning by posting the fire department access number next to each of your telephones. (See Appendix B, the Emergency Information Chart.) Next, make a map of your home and plot out at least two ways to escape the building from every room. It's a good idea to add to your map the location of your fire extinguishers, your first aid kit, and utility cutoffs. You may want to use portable fire ladders from upper floors as part of your plan. If so, practice using them. If you live in an apartment building, your escape routes should take you down stairs, not elevators — an elevator could take you right to the fire.

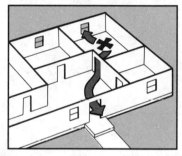

Plot two ways to escape from every room in a fire.

Now practice a fire drill and walk through both of your escape routes. Make sure any locks or latches on your windows and doors open easily from the inside. Since smoke rises during an actual fire, practice crawling close to the ground where the air will be better. Practice this fire drill at least twice a year.

As you work out your family escape routes, decide upon a safe meeting place outside that is far enough away from danger — for example, a mailbox down the street or a corner light. It's important to choose a single location so there will be no confusion. Many deaths have occurred when people reentered burning buildings in order to save missing family members who were in fact outside on the other side of the house.

Should a neighbor's house be on fire, you should leave your home and go to a safer place in case the fire should spread.

Teaching Children about Fire Safety

The first rule of fire safety for children is easy: don't start fires. Tell your children to give all matches or cigarette lighters to adults and to take no chances where fire is concerned.

Talk to your children about what they should do during a fire. Teach your child how a smoke detector works and what it sounds like. Tell them that if a fire does break out they should yell, "Fire!" and get out of the house. Impress upon them that hiding under a bed or in the closet is very dangerous. Practice fire drills with them, and walk them through different situations. Teach them that before they open any door, they should touch it to see if it is hot; if a door is hot, they should use another escape route. If the door is cool, they should open it slowly. If there's fire, heat, or heavy smoke on the other side, they should close the door and leave by a window or other safe exit point. Tell them that it is OK to break a window if they have to get out.

Children should also be taught what to do if their clothes catch fire. This is important because their first impulse will be to run; instead they should *stop, drop, roll,* and *cool.* Tell them to *stop* where they are and not to run. Next, *drop* to the ground and cover their face with their hands, then *roll* over and over to smother any flames. *Cool* the burn with water.

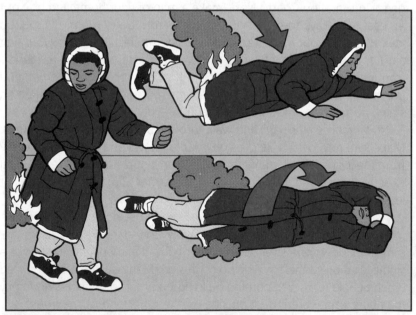

Teach children to *stop, drop,* and *roll* if clothes catch fire.

238   **Part 3: Personal and Family Safety**

You may want to take your children to your fire department to familiarize them with firefighting equipment and procedures. Older children should be taught how to use a fire extinguisher and how to call the fire department from a location outside the house. Tell your children not to worry about their toys or other belongings during a fire, but instead to get out of your home safely.

If a baby-sitter will be taking care of your children, be sure to review fire safety measures with him or her before you go out.

Chapter 7

Disaster Survival

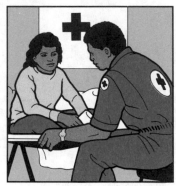

Know which threats might affect your community.

The American Red Cross has been involved in disaster relief since 1881, when Clara Barton, founder of the American Red Cross, organized volunteers and resources to help the people affected by severe forest fires in Michigan. Since that time, the Red Cross has grown into one of the major providers of voluntary disaster relief assistance in the United States. Local Red Cross chapters nationwide also offer a variety of educational materials about how to prepare for and cope with disasters — from natural disasters such as floods to technological disasters such as spills of hazardous materials. During a disaster, trained Red Cross disaster workers meet one-on-one with individuals and families to determine how the Red Cross can help. Local Red Cross workers also set up emergency shelters for those who have lost their homes or have been forced to evacuate.

You can't always prevent a disaster from occurring, but this doesn't mean you're helpless. By familiarizing yourself with the information in this chapter and assembling the recommended supplies ahead of time, you can make sure that you and your family will be well prepared if disaster strikes. Just knowing how to respond to different types of emergencies greatly increases your chances of survival. Having the right supplies can both improve your emergency living conditions and protect your health and safety until normal life resumes.

During a disaster and its aftermath, your top priority is the well-being of your family. It's natural to want to protect your property, but don't take risks trying to save your belongings. If the situation is dangerous, seek safety *immediately*. Then stay where you are until you're certain it's safe to leave. If you have been forced to evacuate your home, don't return to the danger area because you forgot something. And after the immediate disaster is over, don't go sightseeing. You could get in the way of rescue workers as well as expose yourself to dangers such as unstable buildings or downed power lines.

Get Ready

This is a crucial section, but it won't help you if you read it and forget it. After you've reviewed the following information about disaster preparedness, do two things (if you haven't already): make emergency plans and assemble emergency supplies. You'll be able to sleep easier if you do — and if a disaster occurs, you'll be able to respond quickly and effectively with a minimum of anxiety.

What You Need to Know

Before starting your disaster planning, familiarize yourself with the threats that may affect your area. (See box on page 242.) Keep in mind that disasters can occur singly or together. (For example, a hurricane can spawn a tornado, or a severe thunderstorm may cause flash flooding.)

Make sure you and each member of your family knows the name of the county (or, in Louisiana, the parish) in which you live. This way you'll be sure to recognize which emergency bulletins apply to your community. Know in advance whether your area has warning sirens or signals, and which radio or TV stations to listen to during an emergency.

It is important to know the difference between a *watch* and a *warning*. A hurricane *watch*, for example, means that a hurricane may hit your area. A hurricane *warning* means a hurricane is headed for your area so it is time to take immediate action!

Before a disaster strikes, review your homeowner's insurance policy. Policies vary widely when it comes to disaster coverage. If you live in an area that may flood, flood insurance can be an essential investment. You may also want to do a careful inventory of the contents of your home for insurance reimbursement purposes. Keep your important documents as well as your valuables in a safe deposit box.

Making Emergency Plans

There's no substitute for being prepared. Without planning, you magnify the risks of any disaster; but with it, you minimize them. If you have children, be sure to involve them in your planning as well as your safety drills. This will give them a better sense of what to do in an emergency and will help them be less fearful if a real disaster occurs.

After you have made your emergency plans, choose an easy-to-remember day (for example, a birthday or holiday) on which to review them each year.

Which Threats Should You Prepare For?

The following list gives some indication of the threats that might affect your community. If you have any doubt about the kinds of disasters that might occur in your area, contact your local Red Cross chapter for information.

Hurricanes strike coastal areas from Texas to Maine, plus Hawaii, Puerto Rico, and the Virgin Islands. Season: June through November, with peak months August through September. Inland areas may get heavy rains and flooding.

Floods occur all over the United States at any time of year.

Lightning and severe thunderstorms can strike anywhere in the United States at any time of year. They are less common in winter.

Tornadoes have occurred in every state and can occur at any time of year. Peak months: March through August.

Earthquakes can occur in most states at any time without warning. The greatest threat is west of the Rocky Mountains.

Technological disasters and fires can occur in any community at any time.

- *Post a floor plan of your home.* In Chapter 6, you made a floor plan of your home showing escape routes from your home in case of fire. This map should also show the location of your emergency supplies (see page 245) and your home's utility cut-offs (electricity, gas, and water). Post this plan where everyone can see it, and make sure not only your family but also baby-sitters and houseguests understand it.

- *Pick an out-of-state contact.* During a disaster, family members often become separated. Police and emergency workers will be too busy with disaster relief efforts to help you locate members of your family who have taken shelter elsewhere, and it may be impossible for you to make local phone calls. However, you may still be able to place long-distance calls. Choose an out-of-state friend or relative who will act as a central contact who can keep all family members informed. Make sure each member of your family has this person's name, address, and phone number. If you do become separated, call and tell the contact where you are.

- *Choose a meeting place.* It's important to choose a central meeting place that is easily accessible for all members of your family. The understanding should be that you will either (a) unite at this spot if evacuation becomes necessary, or (b) reunite there after a disaster has occurred. It could be a friend's or relative's home or a designated shelter.

- *Practice safety drills.* You already know about fire drills, which were discussed in Chapter 6 and are an essential part of disaster family preparedness. It is also important for you and your family, including children, to practice safety drills for other kinds of natural disasters — for example, a tornado safety drill (head for the lowest spot) or a flood safety drill (head for the highest spot).

- *Prepare your home for an earthquake.* If you live in an earthquake-prone area, there is a great deal you can do to secure the contents of your home in preparation for an earthquake. Earthquakes strike without warning, so it is especially important for you to take safety precautions *now*. Some recommendations:

> Place beds away from windows.
> Place breakable objects in closed cabinets.
> Secure cabinet doors with safety latches.
> Secure heavy mirrors and other large, breakable objects.
> Heavy lamps can be bolted to end tables.
> Store heavy objects on low shelves.
> Strap your hot water heater to the wall.
> Bolt bookcases and other tall, heavy furniture to the wall.

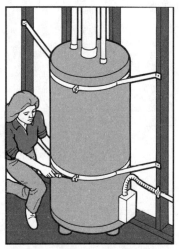

If you live in an earthquake-prone area, be prepared.

Since you can't move far during a serious earthquake — not even across the floor — designate safety spots in each room. (See page 251 for guidelines.)

- *Make an evacuation plan.* If a natural or man-made disaster makes it unsafe for you to stay in your neighborhood, you will be forced to leave your home and seek shelter elsewhere. Local authorities will notify you that evacuation is necessary by sending emergency vehicles with loudspeakers to your neighborhood and/or by sending out the alert over radio or television emergency broadcast systems.

Make an evacuation plan in advance. Decide who will go with whom, and try to stay together in one vehicle. If you live alone, set up a buddy system with a neighbor so you can evacuate together. Discuss what you would do if family members were at work or elsewhere. You may want to keep in mind any relatives or neighbors who are older or disabled and may need special help and decide who will help them.

If you have school-age children, call the school ahead of time

If You Must Evacuate

If evacuation becomes necessary, place the following items in a trash bag, duffel bag, etc.:

- Essential medications (in original containers) for each member of the family (a two-week supply, if possible). To make it easier to obtain refills of prescription medications in the aftermath of the disaster, keep an up-to-date list with the name of each drug plus the name and telephone number of the physician who prescribed it and take it with you.
- A pillow and blanket or sleeping bag for each person
- A change of clothes for each person
- Any necessary aids (for example, canes, walkers, wheelchairs, crutches, dentures, eyeglasses, hearing aids)
- Personal care items (deodorant, toothbrush, toothpaste, etc.)
- Baby supplies (diapers, formula, etc.)
- Favorite activities for each child (books, toys, puzzles)
- Your wallet (including driver's license or identification, credit cards, and money), your checkbook, and your Emergency Information Chart. (See Appendix B.)
- Flashlight and batteries
- Portable radio and extra batteries

Before you walk out the door:

- Put out food and water for your pets. (Health codes don't permit pets in shelters.)
- Write a note explaining where you are going and place it in a prominent place.
- If advised, turn off your utilities (water, gas, electricity).
- Lock up your home.

and find out about its emergency evacuation plan. Then discuss this plan with your children. During a crisis, you might not be able to pick your children up at school or even contact them where they are sheltered. Explain how you will reunite after the disaster is over.

If you do have to evacuate, it's important to leave quickly and early. Pack only emergency supplies (see If You Must Evacuate), and don't worry about your other possessions. Local authorities should inform you of safe routes to take (for example, those that avoid rising flood waters) and should also tell you the location of the nearest shelters.

Emergency Supplies

Now's the time to assemble emergency supplies. These are the things you will need — food, water, and equipment — if you are forced to live at home under emergency conditions. Keep your supplies in a cool, dry place, and check them periodically to make sure that the food is still good, and that the batteries still work. A garbage can with a tight lid makes a good container — it is watertight, can be moved easily, and is itself useful in a disaster.

Some things (for example, fresh food, baked goods, and prescription medications) are difficult to store ahead. As a rule, try to keep two weeks' worth of essential medications on hand at all times just in case your supply is disrupted.

Basic survival supplies to assemble include the following:

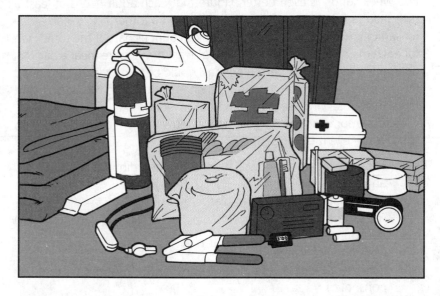

Have emergency supplies ready.

- Battery-operated radio
- Battery-operated flashlight
- Extra batteries
- First aid kit (preferably in addition to the one you have on hand for home use)
- Fire extinguisher
- List with the name of each drug plus the name and number of the physician who prescribed it
- Blanket or sleeping bag for each member of the family
- Watch or battery-operated clock

- Bottled water
- Manual can opener
- Canned food your family likes, packed in water. (Include meats, poultry, fish, fruits, and vegetables for a balanced diet.) Cans are better than jars because they don't break.
- Crackers and cereal. Wrap these in plastic bags and store them in airtight containers to add to their shelf life.
- Foods that store well and do not require cooking (for example, honey, nuts, dried fruit, and chocolate stored in airtight containers or vacuum-sealed)
- Baby food and/or formula and disposable diapers if appropriate
- Pet food as needed

Store at least a three-day supply of food and water for your family. A two-week supply is even better. Figure that each adult needs at least a half gallon of water per day for drinking and another half gallon a day for sanitation. Juice, soup, or other liquids count as part of the total. Plan for each member of the family to eat at least one square meal a day. An optimum allowance per person per day would be two servings of canned meat, poultry, or fish; three to four servings of fruits and vegetables; and three to four servings of cereal and baked goods.

Here are some additional emergency items that are useful to have on hand in the event of a disaster:

- Tape for taping windows; supplies for boarding up windows and doors
- Paper plates and cups and plastic utensils
- Garbage bags
- Toilet paper
- Moistened towelettes
- Personal care items (deodorant, toothbrush, toothpaste, tampons, etc.)
- Clean clothes
- Candles and matches
- Pencil and paper
- A sharp knife
- Needle and thread
- Chemical cold packs
- Tools
- Sturdy shoes
- Rubber gloves

How to Survive a Natural Disaster

In any fight for survival, your three top priorities are shelter, water, and food. In this chapter, you'll learn what to do before severe weather strikes as well as the safest place in which to take shelter during different kinds of natural disasters.

General Guidelines

If the weather in your area is deteriorating, get out your radio and find out what kind of weather is expected. If the National Weather Service issues a weather *watch* for your area, start preparing for severe weather. If it issues a *warning* for your area, this means a natural disaster could occur at any moment. Don't wait for a watch to turn into a warning before taking action. Sometimes there isn't enough time to issue a warning before a disaster occurs.

If you are told to evacuate, do so quickly. If you're at home during a natural disaster:

- Remain calm!
- Grab your emergency supplies.
- Head for the safest place.
- Check everyone for injuries and administer first aid as needed.
- Listen to the radio for updated emergency information.
- Watch out for fire hazards, such as downed power lines or leaking gas. Secondary fires often break out after natural disasters. Check for gas leaks before lighting any matches!
- Eat at least one good meal a day, and drink plenty of water. If you're at home and your power is out, eat food from your refrigerator and freezer first.
- Seal your emergency rations tightly so they will not spoil.
- Stay off the telephone so the lines are clear for emergency calls.

Severe Thunderstorms and Lightning

A severe thunderstorm involves winds over 57 miles per hour or hailstones three-quarters of an inch or greater in diameter. A severe thunderstorm can cause a tornado or flash flood and often knocks out electrical power.

Lightning is always dangerous, whether the accompanying thunderstorm is severe or not. Lightning can start fires and cause electrical injury. Be sure you know how to avoid being struck. (See box on page 248.)

Lightning

Although being struck by lightning is relatively unusual, don't take any chances. Lightning can kill you.

Lightning tends to be attracted to metal, water, and anything tall. With that in mind:

- If you are in a hard-top car (not a convertible), stay there.
- If you are in the water or on a boat, get to shore immediately.
- Avoid masts and metal fixtures.
- If you are outside, seek safety inside a car (not a convertible) or building (not a tent or an isolated shed).
- If you are inside, stay away from the fireplace as well as from open windows and doors. Avoid water (including the bathtub, shower, faucets, or sinks). Stay off the telephone and unplug the television — lightning has been known to travel down electrical wires.
- If you are caught outside and can't find shelter, head for a clump of *short* trees. If you are in the middle of an open field, crouch low to the ground. Make yourself as small a target as possible. Don't lie flat. Kneel or squat (hands on your knees) to minimize your contact points with the ground. If you are in a group of people, spread out. *Stay away* from:

    Hilltops.
    Tall trees.
    Open fields.
    Pools or other bodies of water.
    Evergreens.
    Metal objects (including golf clubs, bicycles, fishing poles, cameras, metal-framed backpacks, tractors, fences).
    Large metal fixtures (flagpoles, ski lifts, utility poles).

Severe thunderstorm watch. A "severe thunderstorm watch" means a severe storm is possible. If the National Weather Service issues a severe thunderstorm watch for your area, take the following steps:

- Be alert for signs that the weather is worsening (for example, storm clouds or darkening skies).
- If you are on the water, head for shore immediately.
- If you are outside, go indoors.

Severe thunderstorm warning. A "severe thunderstorm warning" means a severe thunderstorm will strike soon, possibly within minutes. If the

National Weather Service issues a severe thunderstorm warning for your area, or if you suspect a severe thunderstorm is about to occur:

- Take shelter to avoid being struck by lightning.
- Unplug appliances (computer, television, etc.) so they won't be damaged.

Tornadoes

A tornado is a funnel-shaped cloud spinning at up to 200 miles per hour that moves along the ground destroying everything in its path. Tornadoes can develop from severe thunderstorms or hurricanes and can be accompanied by lightning, heavy rain, and hail. Tornadoes are terrifying, but they pass quickly.

Tornado watch. A "tornado watch" means a tornado is possible. If the National Weather Service issues a tornado watch for your area, stay alert for signs (such as blowing debris or a roaring sound) that a tornado is approaching. Don't wait for an official warning before seeking shelter.

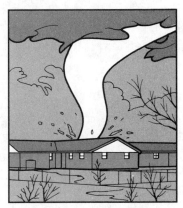

If a tornado watch is issued, stay alert.

Tornado warning. A "tornado warning" means a tornado has been spotted or is about to strike, possibly within minutes. If the National Weather Service issues a tornado warning for your area, or if you see a tornado is approaching, take these precautions:

- If you are outside or in a car, get inside a substantial building (not a tent or mobile home).
- If you are outside and can't get to shelter, lie down in a ditch or low-lying area with your hands over your head.
- If you are inside, stay away from windows. Go to the lowest part of the building — to the basement, if possible. If there is no basement, go to the lowest floor and find an enclosed space (closet, bathroom, hallway) in the center of the building. Get underneath something sturdy and protect your head. If you are in a high-rise building, you may not have time to go to the lowest floor. Pick a place in a hallway in the center of the building.

Floods and Flash Floods

Prolonged rainfall can cause a river to rise until it overflows its banks and causes a flood. This kind of flood develops slowly. Intense rainfall or a break in a dam, levee, or dike can cause a flash flood that strikes with little or no warning.

Flood waters are *dangerous* and may be more powerful than you think. Don't try to walk or drive through flood waters, and don't ignore police barricades.

Flood warning. A "flood warning" means flooding is occurring or will occur soon. If the National Weather Service issues a flood warning for your area:

- Fill the gas tank of your car in case you need to evacuate.
- If you can do so safely, move furniture and valuables to higher ground.
- If your home is likely to be flooded, turn off the utilities (electricity, water, gas).

Flash flood watch. A "flash flood watch" means a flash flood is possible. If the National Weather Service issues a flash flood watch for your area, do the following:

- Be alert for signs of a flash flood (for example, rising flood waters).
- Be ready to evacuate at a moment's notice.
- If you suspect a flash flood, go to safety *immediately*. Don't wait for an official warning before seeking shelter.

Flash flood warning. A "flash flood warning" means a flash flood is occurring. You may have only seconds to escape. If the National Weather Service issues a flash flood warning for your area, or if you suspect a flash flood may occur:

- Leave any low-lying area immediately. Move to higher ground.
- If you are driving in a canyon, get out of your car and climb to higher ground.
- Stay away from streams, creeks, storm drains, and irrigation ditches.

Hurricanes

A hurricane is a huge tropical storm that involves high winds of 74 miles per hour or more, heavy rains, flooding, and sometimes tornadoes. At the center of the hurricane is a calm area called the eye. The most severe part of the hurricane strikes immediately before and after the eye, so don't be deceived by a brief period of calm.

Hurricanes are seldom a surprise. You should have time to get ready and, if necessary, evacuate.

Hurricane watch. A "hurricane watch" means a hurricane is possible. If the National Weather Service issues a hurricane watch for your area:

- Bring in items from outside that may fly around or blow away in strong winds (for example, bikes, lawn furniture, and trash cans).

- Board up windows and doors. Taping windows is an alternative.
- Moor boats securely or move them to safety.
- Turn the temperature control on your refrigerator to the coldest setting before the storm strikes and knocks out your power.
- Make sure you have a supply of fresh water on hand. Fill containers (including the bathtub) now.
- Fill the gas tank of your car in case you have to evacuate.

Hurricane warning. A "hurricane warning" means a hurricane is approaching. Hurricanes travel in an erratic way, so forecasters cannot always predict exactly where a hurricane will hit land. If the National Weather Service issues a hurricane warning for your area, take the following steps:

- If you are told to evacuate, do so quickly. Head inland, since hurricanes weaken over land. Avoid low-lying areas — there may be coastal and inland flooding.
- If you are not told to evacuate, stay inside away from windows. Go to a central part of your home without windows.

Earthquakes

An earthquake causes the ground to shake, move, or even roll. Buildings and bridges can collapse, and power lines can fall. Earthquakes can generate large ocean waves called tsunamis. A large earthquake may be followed by smaller earthquakes, known as aftershocks, which can occur hours, days, weeks, or even months later.

An earthquake usually happens without warning. If you live in an earthquake-prone area, make your house as "earthquake-safe" as possible before an earthquake occurs. (See page 243.) Be alert for early signs of an earthquake, such as glasses rattling, the ground shaking, or a rumbling noise.

If an earthquake strikes:

- If you are inside, immediately go to the nearest safety spot away from windows. Get under something sturdy, such as a desk or a table, and hold onto it, or get into an inside corner of the building.
- If you are caught outside or in your car, stay away from things that might collapse (for example, bridges, buildings, power lines, and trees). If you can, go into an open space. Avoid any structure built on landfill or other soft or unstable soil, and avoid mobile homes.

After a Natural Disaster

The period following a natural disaster can be chaotic and dangerous. It's important to stay out of the way of rescue workers and to let them do their jobs. Don't call the Emergency Medical Services (EMS) system unless there is a real emergency — a serious injury or illness.

Here are some additional guidelines:

- If you are safe and unhurt, stay where you are.
- Stay out of a damaged area until you're certain the situation has stabilized. If you must walk around in a damaged area, wear protective clothing and sturdy shoes and watch out for downed power lines.
- Watch for secondary fires caused by electrical short circuits, overturned space heaters, etc.
- If you're returning to your home, use your flashlight. Check for structural damage. Have the utilities checked and turned back on by a professional. If you smell a gas leak, stay out of the house, make sure the main valve is closed, and notify the gas company. Don't use any electrical appliances that have been in a flooded or wet area.
- Throw out any contaminated or spoiled food.
- Avoid drinking your tap water until local authorities tell you it is safe. If you must drink tap water, boil it first. Your home's water supply may be contaminated because of broken water mains.

How to Survive an Accident Involving Hazardous Materials

"Hazardous materials" is a general term for dangerous substances such as explosives, radioactive waste, flammable gas, toxic fumes, and poisonous chemicals. Many types of potentially hazardous materials pass through our streets and are transported on highways and trains each day. Sometimes industrial or transit accidents or careless disposal of chemicals will release hazardous materials into the environment. Large-scale accidents involving hazardous materials — called "technological disasters" — often force people to evacuate their homes and usually require special cleanup and decontamination procedures.

When accidents involving hazardous materials occur, experienced, knowledgeable personnel must evaluate the site and define the dangers and the extent of contamination. Whether or not evacuation is necessary depends upon the type and amount of the chemical released, how long

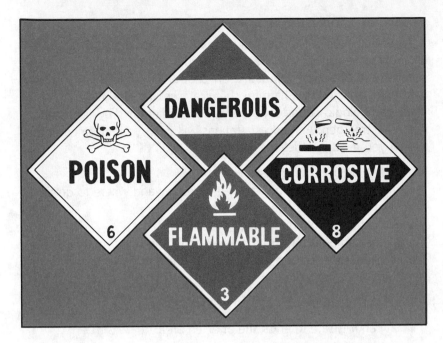

Hazardous materials pass through our communities every day.

it is expected to affect the area, the weather conditions, the time of day, and how long it would take to safely evacuate the area.

Recognizing the Emergency

Hazardous materials can be inhaled, eaten, or absorbed through the skin. You can be exposed to a dangerous substance without realizing because:

- Not all hazardous chemicals can be seen or smelled.
- Some hazardous materials are toxic in tiny quantities that you may not detect.
- Sometimes dangerous substances are not properly labeled.
- You may unknowingly come into contact with something that a hazardous substance has contaminated (for example, clothing, equipment, food, water, or medication).

Accidents involving hazardous materials can be difficult to detect, so be alert to the following danger signs:

- An open or leaking container (for example, a barrel or truck)
- Obvious spillage
- Strange odors or fumes
- Signs and symptoms of poisoning. (See **Poison** on page 163.)

How to Handle the Emergency

Assume that any accident involving a hazardous material is dangerous until it is proven otherwise. Treat any obvious chemical exposure immediately. (See **Chemical Exposure** on page 97.) If you think you may have been exposed to a harmful chemical, seek medical help.

If a technological disaster occurs, you will be notified by local authorities, and emergency broadcast stations will keep you informed. Information you need includes the following:

- The type of health hazard
- Medical treatment that may be necessary and where to get it
- The area that has been affected
- Whether or not you need to evacuate
- If evacuation is necessary, where to go and what routes to take
- If evacuation is not necessary, what precautions to take to minimize your exposure

After the emergency is over, officials should tell you:

- When it is safe to enter the affected area
- Any necessary decontamination procedures
- Signs and symptoms of illness to watch for
- How to seek treatment for chemical exposure

Signs and symptoms of chemical exposure can take time to develop. If you know that you were significantly exposed, or if you are developing any signs and symptoms, consult a physician.

Protecting Yourself During a Chemical Emergency

If you're not directly involved with an accident involving a hazardous substance, stay where you are safe. Don't risk exposure by entering an area that might be contaminated. Stay upwind of the accident so that toxic fumes won't be blown toward you.

Leaving a Contaminated Area

If your community must evacuate because of a technological disaster, you'll be notified by local officials. Gather the essential items you need (see If You Must Evacuate on page 244) and leave as quickly as possible.

If you're in an area where a technological disaster has just occurred, get out of the danger zone immediately. This will minimize your exposure to the hazardous substance.

- If safety officials are present, follow their advice.
- If you're driving through a contaminated area, roll up the win-

dows, close off air vents, and turn off the heat or air conditioning. If possible, cover your nose and mouth with a damp cloth.

- If you are leaving the danger zone on foot, walk so that the wind blows on the side of your face. This way you will walk out of the direct path of the fumes. Don't walk directly into blowing chemicals unless that is the quickest way past the accident.
- Head for high ground and avoid low spots where toxic clouds may settle.

Once you are clear of the contaminated area, avoid contact with others who may not be contaminated. Local authorities will tell you where to go for decontamination.

Sheltering in Place

If you are told by local officials to "shelter in place" rather than evacuate, immediately go inside and seal off your home. Close all windows and doors, turn off the heat or air conditioning, turn off any fans, close any ducts or outside vents (including those to the dryer and stove), and close the fireplace damper. If there is a danger of explosion, close the window shades and curtains, then stay away from the windows.

Next, grab your emergency supplies (see page 245) and go at once to the room with the fewest windows and doors (but avoid the basement, where toxic fumes may settle). Once you are inside this room, seal all gaps — including spaces around doors or windows and any outside vents — with thick tape or wet towels. A wet cloth over your nose and mouth will help filter out dangerous chemicals. Listen to the radio for updates, and stay inside until you are notified that it is safe to leave.

Outdoor and Sports Safety

Sports and outdoor recreation are wonderful, whether your idea of fun is a backyard barbecue, a two-week hike, playing softball, or commuting to work on your bike. In this chapter you will find safety precautions that will protect both your good health and your good times.

Safety Guidelines for Your Yard

Your yard, like anything wild, resists being tamed. You probably spend a good deal of time maintaining it, not only because it is more enjoyable and more beautiful when it is under control, but also because a well-maintained yard is a safer place in which to spend your leisure time.

Some general safety precautions:

- Good outside lighting will help prevent falls and discourage intruders.
- Keep walkways even and free of clutter. In winter, keep sidewalks and steps cleared of ice and snow.
- Store pesticides, insecticides, fertilizer, solvents, and other hazardous substances with extreme care. Store gasoline under lock and key in tightly sealed containers outside your home, away from any potential heat source, and separate from swimming pool chemicals.
- Set up your barbecue in an open area. Avoid lighter fluid, which can flare up suddenly, and dowse all embers when finished. To start a propane gas grill, be sure to light the match *before* you turn on the gas.
- Always wear heavy-duty shoes and long pants when mowing the lawn or using a trimmer. Safety glasses are highly recommended.

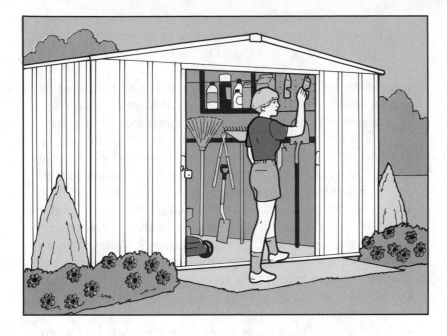

Keep dangerous products and equipment in a locked shed.

- Never mow around children, bystanders, or pets. Even if you have cleared the area, there's still a possibility that objects can be thrown out or that children or pets could slip under the blades.
- Before mowing, clear the area of rocks, sticks, boards, and other debris that could be thrown by the mower blade. Objects can be propelled away from the mower at a speed up to 200 miles per hour.
- Let the lawn mower cool 10 minutes before adding the gasoline to the tank.
- Cover the tops of garden stakes with plastic flowerpots.

Child-proofing Your Yard

It is especially important to child-proof any area where your child spends time alone. It is not enough simply to say, "No." It's good to talk to your child about certain dangers, but keep in mind that he or she may not understand your warnings or may choose to ignore them. If your child is permitted to play by himself or herself in your yard, the area must be child-proofed.

Here is a list of essential precautions:

- Warn your child that outdoor power lines are very dangerous — they carry enough power to kill someone and must never be touched. If a kite becomes entangled in them, leave it alone. If a power line is down or shorting out, don't go near it. Similarly, children should not be allowed to play near electric fences or any other power sources.

- Keep dangerous products and equipment in a locked shed (see also How to Poison-Proof Your Home on page 217). Lock up your gardening tools, ladder, ropes, hoses, lawn mower, trimmer, plastic trash bags, and other potentially dangerous items.
- Check your yard for poisonous plants. (See Poisonous Plants in the next section.) You may want to get rid of the most tempting. Then teach your children which ones are poisonous.
- Get into the habit of scanning the yard for debris and items left behind by other family members before letting a child play.
- Fence any pond or pool. (See also Chapter 9, Water Safety.)
- Never leave a child alone in a yard with a filled swimming pool, even a wading pool. A child can drown in two inches of water.
- Use safety latches on gates so a child cannot let himself or herself through.
- Set up your swing set over a soft surface. Be sure it is properly anchored. Check it frequently for signs of wear, including splinters, frayed ropes, or weak links. Children should use sling seats, not rigid seats. Toddlers should use chair seats.
- Keep sandboxes covered when they are not in use.
- Teach your child never to eat *any* plant without asking an adult.

Poisonous Plants

Plants are tricky. Some are edible; some are not. Some have parts that are nourishing and other parts that are poisonous. For example, the twigs of many fruit trees are poisonous, even though the fruit itself is nutritious. Bulbs, berries, twigs, nuts, leaves, fruit, and seeds or pits can all be poisonous, depending upon the particular plant.

The safest rule is simply to stay away from plants unless you are absolutely certain what they are. Don't touch or eat any plant that you cannot identify. Some very common plants, including houseplants and garden flowers, are toxic, so never assume a plant is benign. Following is a list of poisonous plants. For a list of poisonous plants specific to your area, call your local Poison Control Center. (Note: For how to handle a poisoning emergency, see **Poison** on page 163.)

Many plants are believed to have powerful medicinal qualities, but check with your physician before using a "cure" or preparation recommended by someone who is not a physician.

Certain plants, such as poison ivy, poison oak, and poison sumac, can irritate the skin. How serious the victim's rash will be depends on both the extent of exposure and the individual's sensitivity to the plant.

Common Poisonous Plants

The following plants (or parts of plants) are not safe to eat. If someone you know eats anything on this list, seek advice from your local Poison Control Center.

Flower Garden Plants

Autumn crocus
Bleeding heart
Chrysanthemum
Daffodil
Foxglove
Hyacinth
Iris
Jonquil

Larkspur
Lily of the valley
Morning glory
Narcissus
Poppy
Pothos
Sweet pea

House Plants

Bird of paradise
Castor bean
Dumbcane (dieffenbachia)
English ivy
Holly

Oleander
Philodendron
Poinsettia
Swiss cheese plant

Trees, Shrubs, and Vines

Black locust
Boxwood
Elderberry
English yew
Horse chestnut
Hemlock
Holly (berry)
Hydrangea

Lantana
Mountain laurel
Oak tree
Privet
Rhododendron
Virginia creeper
Wisteria
Yew

Vegetable Garden Plants

Potato (sprouts and other green parts)
Rhubarb (blades)

Tomato (leaves and stems)

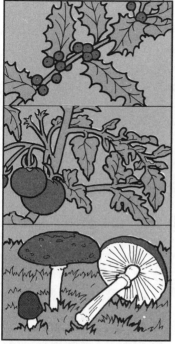

Learn which plants, or parts of plants, are poisonous.

Wild Plants

Bittersweet

Buttercups

Indian tobacco

Jack-in-the-pulpit

Jimson weed

Mayapple

Mescal bean

Mistletoe

Mushroom (some)

Nightshade

Poison hemlock

Poison ivy, oak, sumac

Pokeweed

Skunk cabbage

Water hemlock

Avoiding Bites and Stings

Wherever we live, we're exposed to insects and animals. Most of the time we can peacefully coexist with all kinds of creatures. By following the recommendations in this section, you can keep the peace and minimize your risk of being bitten or stung.

Safety around Animals

Most animals will attack only if provoked. However, never underestimate an animal in its own habitat or an animal that is (or may be) sick. This applies even to your own pet.

To avoid problems:

- Don't provoke any animal.
- Don't disturb an animal that is feeding.
- Don't go near an animal that appears hurt or sick.
- Don't disrupt animals that are mating.
- Don't separate animals that are fighting. If you feel you must interfere, use a long stick.
- If you're camping, don't keep food inside your tent.
- Never feed wild animals.
- Never leave a child alone with an animal, no matter how friendly you believe the animal to be.

If you are threatened by a dog or other hostile animal:

- Don't look the animal in the eye. This may be interpreted by the animal as a threatening gesture.
- Stand still, or back away slowly. Do not run, yell, or make gestures, and do not kick or strike the animal.
- Speak to the animal in a friendly, soothing tone.
- If you are holding food, drop it.

- If the animal clearly is going to bite you, wrap your forearm with a sweater or jacket and hold it out before you.

If the animal does bite your forearm, see if you can block its airway and loosen its grip by pushing your arm against its throat. Do not try to pull your arm away, since this will create a jagged wound. If possible, wait until the animal lets go.

Most animal bites are from pet dogs — man's best friend! A dog is more likely to bite when it's in pain, hungry, frightened, or overexcited. Children should be taught that dogs are not toys. Warn children to be especially cautious around dogs they don't know.

Animal bites can be serious, not only because of the wound itself but also because of the infections that can result. Any bite can cause tetanus, and a bite from a rabid animal can lead to rabies if the victim isn't promptly vaccinated. (For more on animal bites, see **Bites and Stings** on page 50.)

Safety around Snakes

Most of the snakes you may encounter are harmless, but play it safe and avoid all snakes. Snakes are actually shy and will attack only when startled or cornered.

Your best defense against snakes is to know which kinds live in your area or the area you are visiting and to leave them alone. Don't take chances with snakes by approaching or handling them.

Snakes can be found just about everywhere — in the country, in the desert, in the jungle, in rivers or lakes. Find out what the local snakes look like, whether or not they are poisonous, and where you're most likely to encounter them. Snakes are cold-blooded, so when it is cool they seek warmth. In hot weather, they come out at night when it is cooler.

Here are some good general rules to help prevent snakebites.

- When hiking, wear boots and long pants to protect your feet and ankles (the most common target), walk on clear paths, and carry a walking stick.
- Don't reach into an area without looking into it first.
- If you see a snake, stop. Then quickly move at least 20 feet away back along the path you just walked, keeping an eye out for other snakes.
- Don't handle snakes unless you know what you are doing. Remember, even a dead snake can release venom.

Tell children to watch for snakes when they are playing around wood piles, rocks, caves, or other typical snake resting places. Under no circumstances should children be allowed to pick up, play with, or harass snakes.

In North America, there are four kinds of poisonous snakes: the copperhead, coral snake, cottonmouth, and rattlesnake. (See How to Recognize Venomous Snakes in North America on page 56.) Anyone who has been bitten by a poisonous snake needs medical attention immediately (see **Bites and Stings** on page 50). Poisonous snakebites are rarely fatal if prompt medical assistance is obtained. If you are in an area with poisonous snakes and far from medical help, carry a snakebite kit and know how to use it.

Preventing Insect Bites and Stings

There are far more insects in the world than there are people, so chances are good that at some point you will be stung or bitten. Do you know which common poisonous insects are found in your area or in the area you'll be visiting? Could you recognize a scorpion or black widow spider? Could your children?

Most bites and stings are not medical emergencies, but there are exceptions:

- Poisonous bites can be serious. (See How to Recognize Scorpions and Venomous Spiders on page 54.)
- An allergic reaction to a bite or sting can also be serious. For those who are seriously allergic, just one bee sting can be life threatening. Unfortunately, there is no way of knowing whether or not you are allergic until you have a reaction. If you know you are allergic, talk to your physician about carrying an emergency allergy kit with you at all times. (See **Allergic Reaction** on page 45.)
- Multiple stings can be serious if the victim experiences an allergic reaction.
- Certain small pests, including mosquitoes, ticks, and fleas, can transmit a variety of illnesses, some of them potentially serious. (See **Bites and Stings** on page 50.)

To reduce your risk of being stung or bitten while outdoors, follow these general guidelines:

- Wear insect repellent, following the product's application directions. The repellent will last longer if you also apply it to your clothing, but read the package instructions first.
- Avoid wearing perfume, cologne, or aftershave whenever you are planning to spend time outdoors.

- If you're camping, shake out your clothes and shoes before putting them on.
- Cover as much exposed skin as possible. Wear long sleeves, long pants, socks, and a hat. Clothes should be snug at wrists, neck, and ankles. Avoid bright-colored clothes. Keep in mind that insects cannot grab onto slippery cloth (such as nylon) as easily as they can hook into cloth with a loose weave.
- Avoid setting up camp near water or tall, damp grass.
- Learn to recognize and avoid harmful insects and their nests.
- Avoid handling or disturbing any insect, no matter how curious you are or how beautiful it may appear.

If, despite your best efforts, someone is bitten or stung, give first aid promptly and watch for any serious allergic reaction. (See **Bites and Stings** on page 50.)

Hiking and Camping Safety

Hiking and camping provide exercise and interest for everyone of any age. Just getting out and walking around is a wonderful way to see nature. Since unexpected things happen, however, the best way to help guarantee a good time for all is to plan ahead carefully and follow commonsense safety precautions as you travel.

Planning Your Trip

If you have any ongoing medical conditions, it's important to discuss your plans with your physician. Tell your physician where you want to go and get his or her approval first.

Before you go anywhere, mentally walk through your entire hike as you hope it will be. What equipment, supplies, and skills will you need? Write them down. Now walk through your hike again, but this time think it through as you hope it will *not* be. What emergencies could arise? What if you got lost, or were confronted unexpectedly by an animal? What if someone became ill or injured? What kind of weather might you encounter? Add to your list the supplies you would need to deal with these situations. (See box on page 265.)

Before you set out to camp or hike, it's a good idea to read up on the subject as well as take training courses. Make sure you have the skills you may need, from reading a compass or making a temporary shelter to giving first aid. Practice your skills in advance. If your trip will be strenuous, get into good physical condition before you set out. If you plan to climb or travel to high altitudes, make plans for proper acclimatization to the altitude.

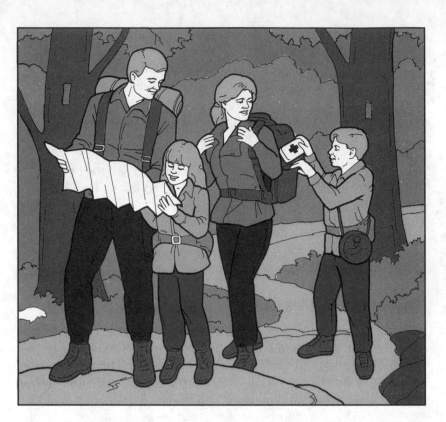

Carry the right equipment when you hike.

Going hiking or camping solo is never a good idea. It's much safer to have at least one companion. If you'll be entering a remote area, your group should have a minimum of four people; this way, if one is hurt, another can stay with the victim while two go for help. If you'll be going into an area that is unfamiliar to you, take along someone who knows the area, or at least speak with those who do, before you set out.

Some areas require you to have reservations or certain permits. If an area is closed, do not go there. Find out in advance about any regulations — there may be rules about campfires or guidelines about wildlife.

If an emergency does occur on your trip, how will you summon help? Pack emergency signaling devices, and know ahead of time the location of the nearest telephone or ranger station.

Once you've worked out your plans, leave a copy of your itinerary with a responsible person. Include such details as the make and year of your car, the equipment you're bringing, and the weather you've anticipated, and, of course, when you plan to return. This way, your contact will have an idea of how well prepared you are in the event that the weather changes or you do not check in on schedule.

What to Bring: A Hiking Checklist

Exactly what you bring will depend upon where you are going and how long you plan to be away, but any well-stocked backpack should include the following:

- Candle
- Clothing. (Always bring something warm, extra socks, and rain gear.)
- Compass
- First aid kit. (See page 6.)
- Food. (Bring extra.)
- Flashlight
- Foil (to use as a cup or signaling device)
- Hat
- Insect repellent
- Map
- Nylon filament
- Pocket knife
- Pocket mirror (to use as a signaling device)
- Prescription glasses (an extra pair)
- Prescription medications for ongoing medical conditions
- Radio with batteries
- Space blanket or a piece of plastic (to use for warmth or shelter)
- Sunglasses
- Sunscreen
- Trash bag (makes an adequate poncho)
- Water
- Waterproof matches, or matches in a waterproof tin
- Water purification tablets
- Whistle (to scare off animals or use as a signaling device)

Always allow for bad weather and for the possibility that you may be forced to spend a night outdoors unexpectedly.

It's a good idea to assemble a separate "survival pack" for each hiker that he or she can keep on his or her person. In a small, waterproof container place a pocket knife, compass, whistle, space blanket, nylon filament, water purification tablets, matches, and candle. With these items, the chances of being able to survive in the wild are greatly improved.

How to Avoid Becoming Dehydrated

Your body needs water — more than you might think — to stay healthy and function correctly. Under extreme conditions or during heavy exertion, your body needs more fluids than usual. You must allow for this and keep your fluid intake in mind as you hike or participate in any strenuous activity.

To avoid becoming dehydrated:

- Drink beyond thirst. Don't rely solely upon your thirst to tell you how much water you need. Thirst can be deceptive, and quenching thirst does not replace all the fluid that is lost under extreme conditions.
- As a precautionary measure, drink six ounces of water every hour while you are hiking, or about four quarts a day.
- Urine should be clear and light colored. If urine output is decreased or if your urine darkens, you need to drink more.
- Avoid coffee, tea, and alcoholic beverages, since they cause fluid loss.

Hiking and Camping with Children

Children love hiking and camping, so by all means take them with you. To ensure that they have a good trip, keep the following safety precautions in mind:

- Before you leave, discuss the possibility of getting lost. Tell children not to wander away. A child who does get lost should call or signal for help if possible, then sit and wait to be found by a search party. The child should hug a tree for security while awaiting rescue.
- Some children panic and hide from rescuers, so mention that this is not a good idea.
- Have children wear something bright so they are easily visible.
- Have children carry a whistle with them to blow if they become lost or frightened. Teach them that a distress signal is three blows on the whistle.
- Warn children not to eat any plants, and teach them to recognize poison ivy.
- Teach children how to avoid bites and stings and how to cope with animals, snakes, and insects.
- Match your pace and the length and difficulty of the hike to the age and skill of the children coming along.

Wilderness Rescue

If you run into trouble in the wild, don't panic. Stay calm. Usually the best course of action is to conserve your strength, send out emergency signals, and wait for help.

An emergency signal can be blowing a whistle, flashing a mirror, lighting a fire, or making a pile of rocks with a message attached. At night, send up a flare or use a flashlight as a beacon.

If you become trapped or lost, search parties may look for you by air. Here are three common ground-to-air signals you might use:

- A large X (this means you're unable to proceed) made with branches, rocks, or extra clothing.
- Three of anything — for example, three flashes of a mirror (this indicates that you are in distress).
- An arrow (to indicate the direction in which you are proceeding).

To attract the attention of air rescuers you, can also make a large design of straight lines in an open field or river bed. Use contrasting colors, or stamp footprints in the snow. Make the design at least eight feet across to be sure it is visible from the air. The color royal blue, which is unusual in nature, is good for attracting attention.

Sports Safety

Exercise is good for you. More and more Americans are realizing that getting up and out is important for both physical and mental well-being. Physical activity performed correctly and regularly benefits your whole body: it conditions the heart and lungs, keeps the joints flexible, improves muscle tone, improves stamina, helps you sleep better and feel more alert, and helps control weight.

Convinced? Good! But before you plunge into a new exercise regimen, have a routine physical examination and get the go-ahead from your physician. This is especially important if you are over 40 and have lived a sedentary lifestyle, or if you're a heavy smoker, overweight, pregnant, or on medication for a long-term health problem.

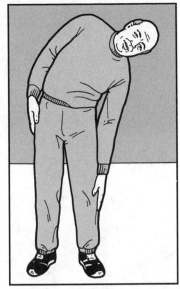

Warm up before you exercise.

How to Prevent Sports Injuries

The most common sports injuries are sprains and strains — injuries to muscles, ligaments, and joints that can be minor or severe. Ordinary muscle stiffness brought on by overexertion heals itself within days, but some sprains and strains are serious and require medical attention.

The human skeleton is draped with over 600 muscles. Most of the time our muscles are uncomplaining, but if you suddenly exert them without proper conditioning or warming up, you may damage them, which leads to pain. To prevent pulled muscles and torn ligaments, heed the following general rules.

- *Warm up first.* A warm-up session before exercising not only helps prevent injuries but can even improve your performance. Warming up starts the blood flowing to the muscles you are about to exert and prepares your body for the physical stress to come.

   Choose a good all-purpose warm-up routine and add any exercises that are necessary for your particular sport. Warm up for at least ten minutes before starting your activity.

   If you have a weak joint, the right exercises can strengthen it. Get professional advice about additional exercises suited to your sport and your particular problem.
- *Cool down afterward.* Don't rest immediately after working out. If you just sit there, even in a hot bath, your muscles will stiffen. Instead, unwind with five or ten minutes of gentle exercise to

bring your pulse closer to its resting rate, then take a quick shower.

- *Get proper training.* If you plan to pursue a sport intensely (which you should, if you want to get any significant benefits), get professional advice. A professional can make sure your technique is proper and advise you if you are doing something that may lead to injury.

  The knees, elbows, and shoulders tend to be most vulnerable because these parts of the body receive unusual use during sports. For example, how many times a day are you aware of your elbow? But what happens as soon as you pick up a tennis racquet? Suddenly your elbow is experiencing a lot of stress. If you condition your muscles carefully, keep a close eye on your form, and take care not to overexert yourself, your elbow will become accustomed to the exertion.

- *Buy the right equipment and clothing.* What equipment and clothing you need depends upon the sport you have selected, but good general rules are to get the advice of a professional before buying anything and to buy quality goods.

  The correct footgear is very important. Wear shoes that fit perfectly and are designed specifically for your activity. Do not wear athletic shoes interchangeably; a good jogging shoe, for example, is constructed differently than a tennis shoe. Some people need special inserts for additional arch support, or perhaps customized shoes. Choose white socks that fit snugly and do not slip; this will protect your feet from blisters.

  Women should wear a well-designed sports bra that gives adequate support. A slight bounce that is not painful indicates a proper fit.

  Research suggests that fluorescent colors (hot pink, lime green) are the safest to wear when exercising outside. Even in broad daylight, people have more trouble spotting blue or yellow clothing. If you will be jogging or bicycling in traffic, you want to be conspicuous!

- *Exercise regularly.* A moderate amount of exercise spread throughout the week is much better for your body than a lot of exertion all at once. Fewer injuries occur to people who condition themselves properly by exercising at least three times a week.

  If you are just beginning to get in shape, exercise until you are sweaty and breathing hard, but not to the point of exhaustion. If your muscles are sore the next day, you have pushed your body too far. Build up your endurance gradually. Many injuries occur when people attempt to do too much too soon.

- *Follow the rules.* Many sports injuries are associated with plain foolishness — people ignoring the warnings on ski slopes, for example, or swimming beyond a safe range. Stick to the rules or restrictions that apply to the area in which you are exercising and to the activity you have chosen.

- *Heed the warnings of your body.* If you experience pain or other limitations during any physical activity, listen to your body — stop and rest. Further exercise at this point could cause damage. If it is still painful to exercise after five minutes of rest, stop for the day and evaluate the problem. Don't apply heat to the affected area or soak in hot water; heat is *not* the correct treatment for sprains, strains, or broken bones. Instead, apply cold packs and elevate the injured area. Cold will reduce swelling if it is applied promptly, and the longer you apply it, the less swelling you're likely to have. (For more on treating sports injuries, see **Bone, Joint and Muscle Injuries** on page 69.)

Long-term injuries may first show up as aches and pains during exercise. As more damage is done over time, the pain and weakness last longer. You need to rest the affected area, and you may need to get medical treatment. Unless the injury is allowed to fully heal, the slightest exertion may cause pain.

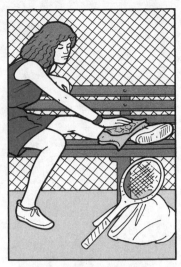

Pain while exercising? Stop and rest. Cold packs are best for swelling.

How to Prevent Sports Injuries in Children

Children are never too young to exercise. Young children seem to run constantly as they develop and strengthen their bodies. Older children often become interested in an individual or team sport. Whatever your child's sports activity happens to be, there are safety precautions to keep in mind.

- Make sure that children have a safe area in which to play. Check your yard, the park, or the playing field for rocks, ditches, holes, torn fences, or other hazards.

- Adequate supervision is essential for children of any age. Guidance from a knowledgeable professional can prevent many injuries. A good coach or trainer always puts player safety first.

- Make sure your child has good equipment that is the right size and that children use their equipment properly.

- Be prepared for a medical emergency. A first aid kit should be on hand, and the players should have access to a telephone and transportation in case an emergency occurs.

- Children tend to suffer sports injuries when the competition becomes too intense. Exercise, fitness, and sports are supposed to be fun; if your child feels he or she has to win at any price, injuries are more likely to occur.
- Children who are not genuinely interested in a given sport are more likely to be injured while playing it. Think twice before pushing your child to participate in a particular sport if he or she is less than enthusiastic about it.
- Teenagers need a pretraining physical examination. The physician will look for anything that could affect or be aggravated by participating in a sport, such as orthopedic and other health problems or growth conditions.

Bicycle Safety

Remember the day you looked back and realized that no one was holding your bike — that you were balancing all by yourself? That day, you probably told the world that you had learned to ride your bike. You weren't quite right, though, because there's much more to learn about riding a bicycle than staying on!

A bicycle is a vehicle, just like an automobile. To ride one safely, you need to know not only how to balance, but how to avoid the situations in which injuries often occur. More and more adults are riding bicycles, and many of them are following outdated or incorrect "rules of the road" they learned in their youth. Bicycles are, in fact, generally subject to the same laws as other vehicles.

The following tips will help you become a safer bike rider:

- *Be predictable.* That means obeying traffic signals, road signs, and pavement signs — just like the other vehicles. When you follow the rules of the road, other drivers will be better able to predict your course.
- *Wear a helmet.* Riding a bike without a helmet is like driving without a seat belt — it just doesn't make sense, especially when you consider that up to 85 percent of serious or fatal bike injuries are the result of head injuries.
- *Be visible.* Your bike is smaller than the other vehicles on the road, so you need to work harder to make yourself seen. Make sure you are riding where drivers would expect to see you. Wear light, bright clothing and a white helmet.
- *Turn, look, and signal.* Before you start a turn, turn your head and look behind you. Then give the proper turn signal. (It's a

good idea to signal when you're about to stop, too.) Give the signal at least 100 feet ahead of your move.

- *Watch out for intersections.* Most bike-car accidents happen at intersections — not just stoplights, but also cross streets and entrances to streets and driveways. Drive defensively and courteously, and try not to confuse other drivers by being timid.
- *Be prepared to yield the right of way,* especially when approaching or passing other cyclists or pedestrians.
- *Don't ride at night.* Children should never be permitted to ride bikes at night. Adults who must ride at night should wear reflective clothing (such as a vest with reflective strips), use a white bike headlight visible from 500 feet, and have reflectors on the bicycle, including a large red rear reflector. Battery-operated blinking lights are available now.
- *Don't pass cars on the right.* It's dangerous, and often illegal.
- *Avoid falls.* Falls are the most common cause of bike injuries — even adults can easily fall off a bike. To avoid falls, use a smooth, consistent routine when stopping and starting. Use care when turning. Keep an eye out for bad pavement, sand, and debris. If necessary, secure your pant legs so they won't get caught in the chain — rubber bands work fine.

Bicycle Safety for Children

Make sure your child's bicycle is the right size. It's tempting to buy a larger bike that will last for years, but it's dangerous for a child to ride a bike that's too big. Make sure your child can straddle the frame with both feet flat on the ground. Young children need a bike with foot brakes because hand brakes require more coordination and strength than many children have. Try to see that broken bicycles are repaired promptly so your children won't be tempted to cruise on an unsafe bike.

Add safety equipment — a chain guard, reflectors, a bell, an orange safety flag, and a basket in the rear if your child needs one. (Front baskets throw off steering.) And make sure your child carries some form of identification, including name and phone number, and that the bike is labeled with the same information.

Children under age nine should not be allowed to ride a bike in the street, but it is never too early to begin to teach your child bike safety, including how traffic works. As you drive, you can educate your child about the meaning of traffic signs and signals, about basic right-of-way situations, and about the difficulties drivers have in seeing cyclists.

As your child grows, teach him or her the general safety guidelines

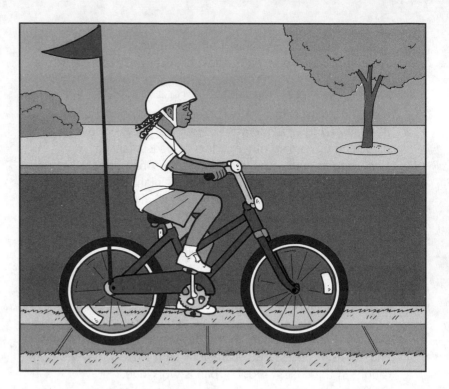

The right bike safety equipment includes a helmet.

above, but all children need to know the following basic bike safety rules:

- *Wear a helmet.* Make sure your child wears a helmet at all times when on a bike or trike. The helmet should have a label showing ANSI or Snell approval. Let the child help pick out the helmet so you'll be sure it's comfortable. And be sure to be a good role model by wearing your own helmet.
- *Walk the bike down the driveway.* Never let your child ride a bike into the street from a driveway — this practice is the most common cause of bicycle accidents for children. Teach your child to walk the bike to the street edge; look left, right, and left until the way is clear; then mount the bike, looking left, right, and left again before proceeding.
- *Look before you turn or swerve.* Another common cause of child bicycle accidents is turning or swerving into traffic. Make sure your child knows that he or she should always look back before turning or swerving.
- *Don't ride at night.* A child's sense of speed and movement is not well enough developed to permit him or her to safely ride a

bike at night. Make children understand that if they are out past sunset, they must get a ride home or walk their bike.

- *Don't ride a bike that's in bad repair.* Instruct your child to let you know if anything goes wrong with a bike. Get your child to help you perform a monthly safety check. Make sure the handlebars, seat, and wheels are tight. Check the brakes and be sure pedals are intact and turn evenly. Spin the wheels — they should not wobble or rub. Get a floor pump and teach your child how to use it to keep the bike's tires inflated. (Once a week is not too often to check tire inflation.)

Water Safety

Millions of Americans enjoy the water and all it has to offer — swimming, boating, fishing, snorkeling, even ice skating. Few things are more refreshing than a quick swim, more invigorating than sailing in a fresh breeze, or more peaceful than a quiet row.

To enjoy the full benefits of water recreation, it's important to know about the kinds of accidents that happen in and around the water and how you and your family can avoid them. It's also important to learn how to participate in the water sport of your choice by taking a course from a qualified instructor. The Red Cross and other organizations offer a wide variety of courses in everything from basic water safety and swimming to kayaking and sailing.

Even if you are an experienced hand around the water, the following sections will help you keep safe.

Swimming

Many excellent swimmers drown, usually because they take unnecessary or unwise risks. Following the correct water safety guidelines is more important than your strength as a swimmer. Whether you are swimming in a pool, pond, lake, river, or ocean, there are certain basic guidelines that always apply.

Basic Safety Guidelines for Swimming

- Learn to swim safely. Classes are available for swimmers of all ages — take one.
- Never swim alone.
- Never swim in unknown waters.
- If possible, swim in areas supervised by lifeguards. Follow their

instructions and respect their judgment. Remember, however, that you share with the lifeguard responsibility for supervising your children.

- Never drink alcohol or use drugs while you are in or around water.
- Don't chew gum or eat as you swim; you could easily choke.
- If you are planning to swim in a new area, check it out first. Each swimming area has its own potential hazards. Swim only when you know the depth of the water and the condition of the bottom. Find out what the water temperature is, whether or not there are dangerous currents or submerged objects, and if there is any dangerous aquatic life.
- Know your limits. If you're not a strong swimmer, stay close to shore or the edge of the pool or shore so you can get to safety by yourself. Don't attempt to keep up with stronger swimmers. Wear a personal flotation device (PFD). (See box on page 278.)
- Respect the limits of others. If you're a strong swimmer, don't tempt others who may not be able to keep up with you. Keep within a safe distance of shore.
- Wear goggles only for surface swimming, not underwater.
- If you have long hair, tie it back or wear a bathing cap — it could get caught underwater.
- Watch out for the dangerous "too's" — too overheated, too cold, too tired, too far from safety, too much sun.
- Be alert for warning markers and heed them.
- If stormy weather is approaching, get out of the water.
- Don't swim in very cold water.
- Don't swim in polluted water.
- Always keep an eye on younger swimmers.
- Don't horse around. This includes:
     No running around a pool
     No pushing
     No jumping on others in the water
     No dunking
     No diving or jumping into shallow water
     No screaming or faking emergencies

If you follow all of these guidelines, you shouldn't run into problems. If you do, however, the first rule is to *stay calm*. Panicking will only place you in greater danger. If you need to signal for help, wave one arm as high above your head as you can.

- *If you get a cramp*, try to stretch it out while floating in the water. Then swim to safety, if possible using a different stroke than you were using before.

- *If you become exhausted*, float until you feel rested.
- *If you are caught in a current*, swim across it, not directly against it.

(*Note:* For water rescue, see **Drowning** on page 121.)

Keeping Children Safe in and around the Water

The following safety guidelines apply whenever children are around water, whether you are at a public beach or pool or in the backyard.

- Enroll your child in water safety and swimming courses.
- If for any reason you discover your child is missing, check the water first.
- *Never* leave a child alone near water, even for a second. This is true even if the child has had swimming lessons or is wearing a personal flotation device (PFD). Keep your eyes on the child, and don't leave to answer the phone or the door.
- Restrict young children to shallow water, where their feet can touch bottom.

Enroll your child in water safety and swimming courses.

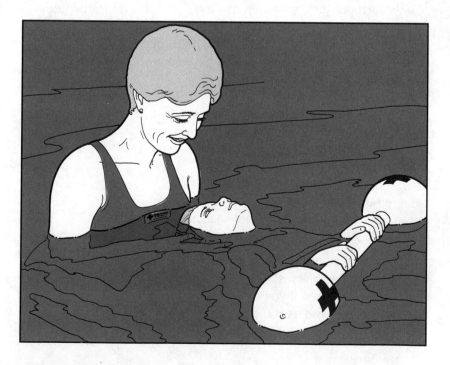

- If more than one adult is keeping an eye on the kids, be very clear about which adult is watching which child. Children have drowned when one adult assumed another was watching.
- If the pool or beach is unfamiliar, get in the water yourself and check out the slope of the bottom, how slippery it is, how deep the water is, and whether or not there are any sudden drop-offs.
- Be sure your baby-sitter knows how to swim. The baby-sitter should also be familiar with the place where children are swimming and know the pool or beach rules.
- Don't rely on flotation devices to keep a child safe. They can give a child a false sense of security, and suddenly he or she will be in over his head — literally.
- Don't permit horseplay.
- At the beach, keep an eye on tides; water can quickly reach children building sand castles, etc.

Private Swimming Pools

If you own your own pool, the number one safety precaution is to enclose it on all four sides. Even if you have no children of your own, don't run the risk of having neighboring children fall in, or of having others invite themselves for a swim in your absence.

Many states and counties have regulations concerning pool fences. If yours doesn't, or isn't specific, choose a fence that is at least five feet high on all sides. If there are horizontal supports, make sure they are on the inside so children cannot use them to climb over the fence. The spaces between vertical slats should be less than four inches. Use a gate that swings shut and latches automatically. Make sure the latch is out of the reach of children, and lock the gate when the pool is not in use.

If one side of your pool enclosure is your house, you *must* take precautions to avoid unwanted access to your pool from the house. Any doors or windows must be locked in a way that prevents children from getting to the pool. Otherwise, a momentary lapse in supervision could lead to tragedy.

Consider putting an alarm on the gate to the pool and a pool alarm in the water. Pool alarms are devices that go off whenever there is sound or a change in pressure below the surface of the water. If anything heavy falls in, the alarm will sound.

What else should you do?

Personal Flotation Devices (PFDs)

A *personal flotation device* is something designed to keep you from sinking when you are in or around water. There are five basic kinds of PFDs, and there is one that is appropriate for every type of water activity, from swimming to boating to water sports. They include life preservers, buoyant vests, special-purpose devices for water recreation, buoyant cushions, and ring buoys. *PFDs save lives.*

Choose a Coast Guard–approved PFD appropriate for the activity you're engaged in. Make sure it's the proper size and that you can swim in it. Remember that when boating, you must have a PFD for every person on the boat.

- If you have an above-ground pool, remove the steps when the pool is not in use.
- Use dividing ropes to designate sloping areas.
- Keep the water level three inches from the top of the pool so a child can hang on to the edge and breathe.
- Properly mark the depth of the water.
- Don't permit diving in water less than 9 feet deep or in above-ground pools.
- Keep the pool covered during the off-season.
- Completely remove the pool cover when the pool is in use.
- Be sure that steps leading from the pool have handrails.
- Install a nonslip surface around the edge of the pool.
- Keep toys out of the pool when not in use — they're a nuisance and can attract the attention of children.
- Keep a first aid kit in the pool area.
- Keep a phone in the pool area.
- Post emergency phone numbers (see Appendix B) and the tear-out Emergency Action Guides from this book in a prominent area where they will not get wet.
- Have a life ring with a line attached and a hooked pole (preferably one that floats) close at hand.
- Take courses in CPR and water safety. If you have children, take an infant-and-child CPR course.
- Have nighttime lighting in case of emergency.
- Don't allow glass or electrical appliances in the pool area.
- Properly store and lock pool chemicals. Don't store them near gasoline.

Swimming in Ponds, Lakes, and Rivers

If you live on a body of water that's suitable for swimming, keep the same rescue devices on hand as you would for a pool. Mark off a safe area in which to swim, and post signs for danger areas.

If you plan to swim in an unfamiliar pond or lake, check the bottom first. Walk in carefully the first time you enter. Watch for hidden rocks or branches as well as large clumps of water weeds. If there are boats in the area, attempt to mark off your swimming area and watch out for passing motorboats and fishing lines.

Like lakes, rivers can have submerged rocks, fallen trees, or other hidden obstacles. Another concern is the current. Stay out of fast-moving water. If you find yourself caught in a swift current, roll onto your back and let the current take you downstream, feet first. When you are out of the swift current, swim downstream while angling toward the shore.

Ocean Swimming

Ocean swimming is not at all like freshwater swimming. Because of the constant pounding of the waves, swimming in the ocean is more physically demanding. Currents and bottom conditions can also be tricky, so do some research before you swim. Find out if there are any undertows that could pull you away from shore. Ask how strong the tides are, and check for sudden drop-offs underfoot.

If the waves are strong enough to knock you over, stay close to shore, where you have firm footing. If a large wave suddenly comes along, it's far easier to duck under it than to fight it. Use your judgment about letting small children play in the surf.

If you want to take a long swim, don't swim straight out from shore. Instead, swim parallel to the shore. Do not swim out with a current, or float out on a raft; you may find that you cannot swim back to shore again. If you start to swim and discover an undertow is carrying you away from shore, swim parallel to the shore until you are clear of the current. Then swim back to shore.

Be alert for dangerous marine life. A wide variety of poisonous creatures live in the ocean. Some have far-reaching tentacles, some have spines; and while many are beautiful, they are also capable of stinging you and releasing harmful venom. In some areas, sharks are a problem. Take the time to learn to recognize the marine life you may encounter, and heed all posted warnings on beaches concerning marine life. If you find yourself close to an unwelcome creature, move away as cautiously as possible.

Chapter 10

Auto Safety

Driving is such a routine part of our lives that most of us don't think much about it. It's easy to forget that when you drive a car, you are in fact commanding thousands of pounds of steel at high speeds under unpredictable circumstances.

Whether you are going around the block or across the country, ask yourself two questions before you get behind the wheel of your car or any other vehicle:

1. *Am I in shape to drive?* Before going anywhere, make sure you feel rested and fit. Fatigue, medications, and drugs, including alcohol, can inhibit your ability to stay alert and respond quickly. If you are tired, angry, or under the influence of alcohol or any other drug, *don't drive.* It can't be said too often: *Drinking and driving kills!*

2. *Is my car in shape to be driven?* An unsafe car can kill you. Make sure your car is always properly tuned and in good working condition. Check the condition of the tires, the tire pressure, and the brakes routinely, as well as fluid levels — antifreeze, oil, and brake fluid. While you're at it, check your mirrors, clean your windshield wiper blades, and top off the washer fluid reservoir. The temperature controls should be able to keep the interior of the car comfortable and the windows defrosted. Be sure your spare tire is inflated. Also keep in mind that your car isn't ready to be driven until you have packed the right emergency equipment. (See box on page 283.)

Before you turn on the ignition, put on your glasses or sunglasses if you need them and BUCKLE UP. As specialists have concluded from actual crash data, buckling up is the simplest, and probably the most effective, protection against serious injury or death. If everyone buckled up, the severity of several million personal injuries a year would be reduced. It has already been said a million times, but it bears repeating: *seat belts save lives*.

If you're buying a car, seriously consider one equipped with air bags. And, of course, once you start the car, drive safely and defensively.

Driving with Children

Everyone, regardless of age and no matter how short the trip, needs a safety restraint. Don't set out until every passenger is buckled up. Since children are small, they are at greater risk for being thrown around the inside of the car or thrown from it during an accident.

Older children should sit in the backseat with seat belts fastened. Infants and young children need special car seats because their bodies are not developed enough to withstand the pressure of an ordinary seat belt if a car crash occurs. Make sure children are secured in federally approved child seats each time they go out in a car. If your child will be traveling in someone else's car, send the seat along. Be sure, too, to secure the safety seat to the seat of the car. Holding a child on your lap is *not* safe. Even if you are wearing your seat belt, the child could catapult out of your arms. If you've fastened the child in your lap with the safety belt, your child could be crushed by your weight in an accident.

- An *infant seat* is needed for babies of up to about 20 pounds. These bucket-shaped seats face the rear of the car. If an accident occurs, the force of the impact will throw the baby's back against the protective seat. (A baby's chest and abdomen are too delicate for other types of restraints.)
- A *car seat* is appropriate for children of about 20 to 40 pounds. Car seats face the front and have a harness or shield or combination of both.
- A *booster seat* (designed for car use) is for children of about 30 to 60 pounds.

Other safety guidelines for driving with children:

- The back seat is safer than the front seat.
- Never leave children unattended in the car.
- Until children reach about age six, use safety locks on the rear doors so they cannot let themselves out unexpectedly.
- Always feel a car seat to make sure it's not too hot before putting a child in it.

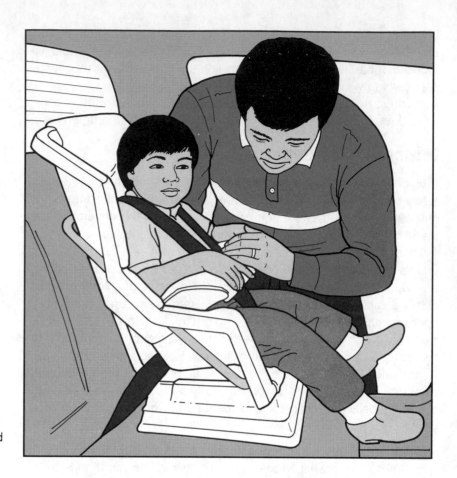

Make sure children are secured in a car safety seat.

- Look out for fingers when closing doors.
- Lock automatic windows.
- Riding in the cargo area of a van or station wagon without seat belts is unsafe.
- Never permit children to ride in the bed of a truck, even if the truck has a cap.
- When letting children out of the car, open the door at curbside, not into the street.
- Make sure all articles within the car are put away. During an accident, anything that is loose — tissue boxes, pencils, even pieces of toys — can become a serious hazard.
- Be sure there are no sharp objects protruding anywhere. (This includes pockets!)

Emergency Supplies for Your Car

You probably have a jack in the trunk of your car — you should. But the following emergency equipment should also be kept in your car or other vehicle, particularly for an extended trip or when driving in extreme weather conditions. If you run into trouble on the road, these items may become your survival supplies. You won't use them often — but when you need them, you'll be glad you brought them. Most of these items are not expensive, but you need not go out and buy brand-new ones if you already have supplies on hand that are in good condition.

In a large sturdy plastic bag, put:

Blanket
Dehydrated food
Electrical tape
Emergency flares or emergency triangular reflector
Fan belt (spare)
Fire extinguisher. (Use a BC type — see page 236.)
First aid kit. (See page 6.)
Flashlight (or another light source) and batteries
Gas siphon
Ice scraper
Jumper cables
Repair wire
Road atlas
Rope (16 feet of nylon clothesline)
Sharp scissors
Shovel
Tool kit (including tools for changing a flat tire, wire cutters, and screwdrivers)
Trunk tie-down
Water bag or flexible container
Waterproof matches

Taking Car Trips

Long trips by car will be safer and more enjoyable if you are well rested and allow plenty of time to reach your destination. To help keep alert, eat lightly and make frequent stops. Wear loose clothing. If car sickness is a problem, you can help reduce nausea by looking straight ahead (instead of out the side windows) and into the distance (instead of close up). Since over-the-counter anti-nausea medications can make you sleepy, don't take them if you will be driving. Consult your physician if necessary.

Auto Travel in Severe Weather

In emergencies, people often stay with or abandon their automobiles at the wrong time. Listen to the radio for the latest National Weather Service bulletins on severe weather for the area in which you drive. Try to find out the name of the county (or in Louisiana, parish) in which you are driving because weather advisories are issued by county. Stay informed as forecasts change. Following are some safety tips for motorists in various types of emergencies. In any situation, the most important rule is to *remain calm*.

Blizzard

Winter travelers should be prepared to spend the night in the car. If you're caught in a storm and your car is immobilized, stay in the car. Don't try to walk from your car unless you can see a safer haven close by. If you are stranded, turn on the engine for brief periods to provide heat, leaving a window slightly open to avoid poisoning from fumes. Make sure the exhaust pipe is clear of snow. Do not remain in one position for a long time; a form of mild exercise is best. Leave the dome light on at night as a signal if the flashers are buried in snow. If more than one person is involved, sleep in shifts.

Tornado

If a tornado warning has been issued, seek safety in a substantial building. If you see a tornado and there is no structure nearby, get out of your car and lie flat on the ground in a ditch with your hands over your head.

Hurricane

Evacuate early if you are told to do so. Keep a full tank of gas during the hurricane season and learn the best evacuation route from your home, your place of work, and the area where you are traveling. Head inland and avoid low-lying areas — the most dangerous part of a hurricane is the coastal flooding (called *storm surge*) it causes.

Flood

If you are told to evacuate, do so immediately. If you come upon flood water, abandon your car and climb to higher ground. If the car stalls in water, get out and quickly move to higher ground. Flood waters rise rapidly, and a car can be swept away. Never drive through water on a flood zone road; the water can be deeper than it appears. Observe barricades and other warnings.

Earthquake

Stop the car away from buildings, power lines, or trees. Stay in the car until shaking stops. The car's suspension will cause the car to shake violently during an earthquake, but it is still a safe place to be. Continue on your way after the shaking stops, avoiding bridges, underpasses, and other structures that may have been damaged by the quake or could be damaged further by aftershocks.

Thunderstorm

Your car is one of the safest places to be in a thunderstorm, as long as it is not a convertible. Turn the radio off. If there is poor visibility, pull to the side of the road until conditions clear. If you do need to pull off the road, avoid parking under power lines or next to large trees, tall poles, and other things that may attract lightning or blow down during high winds.

Breakdowns

No matter how well you plan, tires do go flat and cars do break down. If this should happen to you:

- Pull well off the road.
- Put on your car's blinking hazard lights.
- Put up your car's hood.
- Set up flares and/or your emergency reflective triangle.
- If necessary, warn traffic away from your car, but *don't endanger yourself*.
- Get help if help is nearby. If you can't see where to get help, stay with your car.

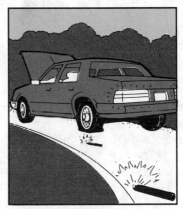

Pull well off the road, turn on hazard lights, raise the hood, and set flares.

What to Do if You Are Involved in a Car Accident

If you are involved in a car accident but are *unhurt*, take the following steps:

- Stop the car. Turn off the ignition and set the hand brake.
- If injuries have occurred or are suspected, have someone call EMS as soon as possible. Give first aid.
- Don't move any vehicle until police arrive and advise you to do so.
- Name, address, phone number, vehicle registration, and insurance information should be obtained from all motorists involved.
- It may be a good idea to find an independent witness (someone

who was not traveling with you) who will be willing to make a statement regarding the accident later.

Car accidents are very frightening, and emotions can run high. Try to remain calm. Whatever the circumstances may be, this is not the time to become argumentative or resentful.

If you *are injured*, don't push yourself. Let others help you, and try to remain calm as you wait for EMS.

Pedestrian Safety

When you're driving, be on the lookout for pedestrians — and when you are on foot, watch out for cars! Look and listen closely. Don't wear a headset when you walk, jog, or bicycle near traffic. Wait for traffic lights to be in your favor and allow enough time to cross safely.

Pedestrian Safety Guidelines for Children

Children are especially at risk around traffic. They cannot understand all the complexities of a given situation and are not aware of all the unpredictable moves a vehicle may make. They aren't experienced at judging distance or speed, and they don't realize how long it can take a car to come to a stop — or that under certain conditions, drivers simply can't see them.

Tell your child to stop, look both ways — left, then right, then left — and listen before crossing a street. Teach him or her the meaning of traffic signs. Warn your child that a green light does not necessarily mean it is safe to cross.

Other safety tips for children include the following:

- Never run into the street.
- Never stand or walk between parked cars.
- Don't cross the street in the middle of a block. Always use crosswalks.
- Be especially careful when it's hard to see well — such as at dusk and after dark or in rain, fog, snow, or bright sun.
- Watch out for blind curves (bends in the road that neither a driver nor pedestrian can see around).
- Walk on the sidewalk facing traffic. If there is no sidewalk, walk on the edge of the road facing traffic.
- Stay 10 feet from the front of a bus or truck that is parked, and never walk behind either. Bus and truck drivers are seated up high and cannot see children on the ground directly in front of or behind their vehicles.

Appendixes

The appendixes and the Emergency Action Guides are designed to be pulled out of the book and copied as needed.

Appendix A: First Aid Kit Checklist

Put a copy of this in your first aid kit. Once a month, use it to review your kit and then replenish and replace supplies as needed.

Appendix B: Emergency Information Chart

Fill out copies of the form for your home and workplace. Then post them near telephones, and put one in your first aid kit. They will prepare you to give important information to an EMS dispatcher in an emergency situation.

Appendix C: Consent and Contact Form

Fill out a copy of this form when you leave your child (children) with a caregiver, sitter, or someone else who might have to seek emergency medical care for the child in your absence.

Emergency Action Guides

These are quick references for lifesaving techniques. They cover choking, CPR, and how to control bleeding. Tear them out and post them on your refrigerator, near your desk at work, or wherever you feel you may need them.

First Aid Kit Checklist

☐ Copy of *The American Red Cross First Aid and Safety Handbook*
☐ Filled-out copy of the Emergency Information Chart

Dressings

☐ Adhesive bandage strips
☐ Butterfly bandages
☐ Elastic bandage, 3 inches wide
☐ Hypoallergenic adhesive tape
☐ Roller bandages
☐ Sterile cotton balls
☐ Sterile eye patches
☐ Sterile gauze pads, 4 by 4 inches
☐ Sterile nonstick pads
☐ Triangular bandage

Instruments

☐ Blunt-tipped scissors

☐ Tweezers
☐ Bulb syringe

Equipment

☐ Cotton swabs
☐ Eye cup or small plastic cup
☐ Instant-acting chemical cold packs
☐ Paper cups
☐ Space blanket
☐ Thermometer

Medication

☐ Activated charcoal
☐ Antiseptic wipes or antiseptic solution
☐ Antiseptic/anesthetic ointment or spray
☐ Calamine/antihistamine lotion
☐ Sterile eye wash
☐ Syrup of ipecac

Miscellaneous

☐ Change for pay phone
☐ Candle and matches
☐ Flashlight
☐ Pad and pen or pencil
☐ Packet of tissues
☐ Soap
☐ Safety pin
☐ Disposable latex gloves
☐ _____
☐ _____

Emergency Information Chart

Emergency Telephone Numbers

EMS _____ Fire _____

Poison Control Center _____ Police _____

Ambulance _____ Other _____

Family Physician: Name _____ Phone _____

Nearest Hospital: Name _____ Phone _____

Address _____

_____

Directions _____

_____

When you call EMS, be ready to provide the following information:

Your name _____

Type of emergency _____

Location of emergency _____
street address

_____
apartment number

_____
nearby landmarks

_____
major intersections

Telephone number you're calling from _____

How many are injured? _____

DON'T HANG UP UNTIL THE DISPATCHER TELLS YOU TO!

Consent and Contact Form

This form is to be completed and signed by the parent or legal guardian.

Name(s) of child (children) _____

In the event the child (children) named above is (are) injured or ill, I understand that the caregiver will attempt to contact me, the other parent, or the legal guardian at the telephone number provided below.

Parent's (legal guardian's) name _____

Telephone numbers _____ on _____ (hours/days)

_____ on _____ (hours/days)

Parent's (legal guardian's) name _____

Telephone numbers _____ on _____ (hours/days)

_____ on _____ (hours/days)

In the event that I and the other listed are not available, I give my permission to the caregiver to provide first aid for the child (children) named above and to take the appropriate measures, including contacting the emergency medical services (EMS) system and arranging for transportation to _____

_____

or the nearest emergency medical facility.

Signature _____

Medical Insurance Plan _____

Group Number _____ ID Number _____

CHOKING: ADULT OR CHILD
(Over 1 Year of Age)

American Red Cross

1. Ask If Person Is Choking

- If person can't answer, call EMS. Go to Step 2.
- If person is coughing forcefully and can breathe, do not interfere. Stand by.

2. Position Your Hands

- Wrap your arms around person's waist.
- Make a fist. Place thumb side of fist in middle of person's abdomen (above navel and well below lower tip of breastbone) (Fig. 1 inset).

3. Give Abdominal Thrusts

- Grasp fist with other hand.
- Press fist with quick, upward thrusts into abdomen (Fig. 1). Continue until person either starts breathing or loses consciousness.

IF PERSON IS UNCONSCIOUS

4. Call EMS if Someone Hasn't Already

5. Place Person on Back

- Clear mouth if necessary.
- Check for breathing.
  If no breathing . . .

6. Begin Rescue Breathing

- Tilt head back and lift chin (Fig. 2).
- Pinch nose shut.
- Seal your lips tightly around mouth (Fig. 3).
- Give 2 full breaths for 1 to 1½ seconds each.
  If breaths won't go in . . .

OVER

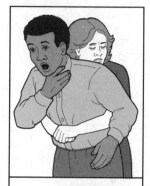
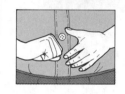

Figure 1

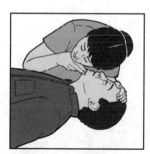

Figure 2

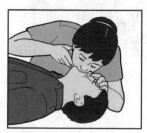

Figure 3

7. Retilt Head and Try Again

- Tilt head farther back.
- Pinch nose shut, seal your lips, and try again to give 2 breaths.
  If breaths still won't go in . . .

8. Give Abdominal Thrusts

- Straddle person's thighs.
- Place heel of hand in middle of abdomen, just above navel and well below lower tip of breastbone.
- Place other hand on top and point fingers toward person's head (Fig. 4).
- Give 6 to 10 quick thrusts inward and upward.

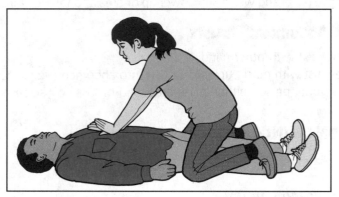

Figure 4

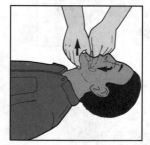

Figure 5

9. Do Finger Sweep

- Grasp tongue and lower jaw. Lift jaw.
- Slide finger down inside cheek to base of tongue (Fig. 5). Sweep object out.
  If person is still not breathing . . .

10. Go Back to Step 6

- Repeat sequence until person begins to cough or breathe.

EMS or emergency phone number_____

CHOKING: INFANT
(Newborn to 1 Year of Age)

American
Red Cross

1. Is Baby Choking?

- If baby can't cough, breathe, or cry, or is coughing weakly, call EMS. Go to Step 2.
- If baby is coughing forcefully and can breathe, do not interfere. Stand by.

2. Turn Baby Facedown

- Hold baby's jaw and support head as you turn baby facedown.
- Rest your forearm on your thigh.

3. Give 4 Back Blows

- Use the heel of your hand.
- Give 4 blows forcefully between shoulder blades (Fig. 1).

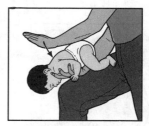

Figure 1

4. Turn Baby onto Back

- Support head.
- Rest baby's back on your thigh.

5. Give 4 Chest Thrusts

- Place index and middle fingers on baby's breastbone, just below nipples (Fig. 2).
- Give 4 quick thrusts down ½ to 1 inch.

6. Go Back to Step 2

- Repeat sequence until baby coughs up object or starts to cough, cry, or breathe.

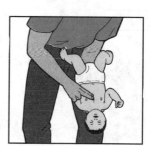

Figure 2

IF BABY IS UNCONSCIOUS

7. Call EMS if Someone Hasn't Already

OVER

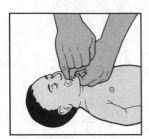

Figure 3

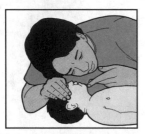

Figure 4

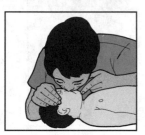

Figure 5

8. Place Baby on Back

- Move baby as a unit. Place on firm surface.

9. Look into Baby's Mouth

- Grasp tongue and lower jaw. Look for object in mouth.
- Sweep any object out with your little finger (Figure 3).

10. Begin Rescue Breathing

- Look. listen, and feel for breathing.
  If no breathing . . .
- Gently tilt head back and lift chin (Fig. 4).
- Seal your lips tightly around nose and mouth (Fig. 5).
- Give 2 slow breaths for 1 to 1½ seconds each.
  If breaths will not go in . . .

11. Retilt Head and Try Again

- Tilt head farther back.
- Seal your lips and try again to give 2 breaths.
  If breaths still won't go in, repeat Steps 2 through 6 until airway is cleared or help arrives.

EMS or emergency phone number_____

CPR: ADULT

1. Check for Consciousness

- Tap or gently shake person.
- Shout, "Are you OK?"

2. Shout, "Help!"

3. Roll Person onto Back

- Move person as a unit. Support head and neck. Place on firm surface.

4. Open Airway and Check Breathing

- Tilt head back. Lift chin (Fig. 1).
- Look, listen, and feel for breathing for 5 seconds.
  If no breathing . . .

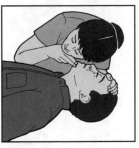

Figure 1

5. Give 2 Full Breaths

- Pinch nose shut.
- Seal your lips tightly around mouth (Fig. 2).
- Give 2 full breaths for 1 to 1½ seconds each.

6. Check Pulse

- Feel for pulse at side of neck for 5 to 10 seconds (Fig. 3).
  If no pulse . . .

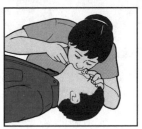

Figure 2

7. Phone EMS for Help

- Send someone to call.

OVER

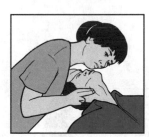

Figure 3

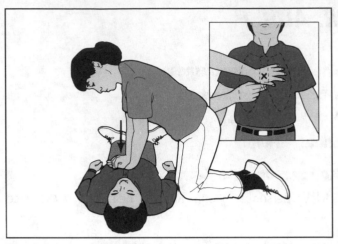

Figure 4

8. Position Your Hands

- Find notch at lower end of breastbone with middle finger.
- Place heel of other hand on breastbone, 2 finger-widths above notch (Fig. 4 inset).
- Remove fingers from notch and place heel of this hand over heel of other hand.
- Keep fingers off chest.

9. Give 15 Compressions

- Lean with shoulders over your hands. Lock your arms (Fig. 4).
- Depress breastbone 1½ to 2 inches.
- Give 15 compressions in 10 seconds.

10. Give 2 Full Breaths

- Tilt head back. Lift chin.
- Pinch nose shut (Fig. 5).
- Give 2 full breaths for 1 to 1½ seconds each.
- Check pulse.
  If no pulse . . .

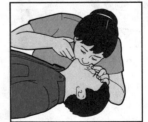

Figure 5

11. Repeat Cycles of 2 Breaths and 15 Compressions for 4 Cycles

- Continue until person revives or help arrives.

EMS or emergency phone number_____

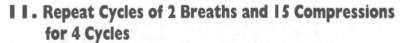

CPR: CHILD
(Age 1 to 8)

1. Check for Consciousness
- Tap or gently shake child.
- Shout, "Are you OK?"

2. Shout, "Help!"

3. Roll Child onto Back
- Move child as a unit. Support head and neck. Place on firm surface.

4. Open Airway and Check Breathing
- Tilt head back. Lift chin (Fig. 1).
- Look, listen, and feel for breathing for 3 to 5 seconds. *If no breathing . . .*

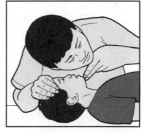

Figure 1

5. Give 2 Slow Breaths
- Pinch nose shut.
- Seal your lips tightly around mouth (Fig. 2).
- Give 2 slow breaths for 1 to 1½ seconds each.

6. Check Pulse
- Use one hand to keep head tilted.
- Feel for pulse at side of neck for 5 to 10 seconds (Fig. 3). *If no pulse . . .*

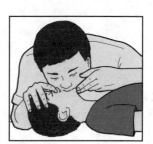

Figure 2

7. Phone EMS for Help
- Send someone to call.

OVER

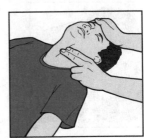

Figure 3

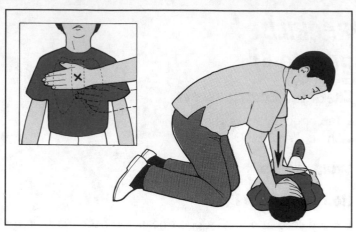

Figure 4

8. Position Your Hands

- Keep head tilted with one hand.
- Find notch at lower end of breastbone with middle finger. Place heel of same hand on breastbone, 2 finger-widths above notch (Fig. 4 inset).
- Keep fingers off chest.

9. Give 5 Compressions

- Lean with shoulder over hand. Lock arm straight (Fig. 4).
- Depress breastbone 1 to 1½ inches.
- Give 5 compressions in about 4 seconds.

10. Give 1 Slow Breath

- Tilt head back. Lift chin.
- Pinch nose shut.
- Give 1 slow breath for 1 to 1½ seconds (Fig. 5).
- Check pulse.
  If no pulse . . .

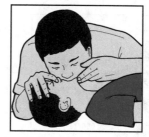

Figure 5

11. Repeat Cycles of 1 Breath and 5 Compressions for 10 Cycles.

- Continue until child revives or help arrives.

EMS or emergency phone number_____

CPR: INFANT
(Birth to Age 1)

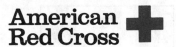
American Red Cross

1. Check for Consciousness
- Tap or gently shake baby's shoulder.

2. Shout, "Help!"

3. Roll Baby onto Back
- Move baby as a unit. Support head and neck. Place on firm surface.

4. Open Airway and Check Breathing
- Gently tilt head back. Lift chin (Fig. 1).
- Look, listen, and feel for breathing for 3 to 5 seconds. *If no breathing . . .*

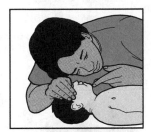
Figure 1

5. Give 2 Slow Breaths
- Seal your lips tightly around nose and mouth (Fig. 2).
- Give 2 slow breaths for 1 to 1½ seconds each.

6. Check Pulse
- Use one hand to keep head tilted.
- Feel for pulse in upper arm for 5 to 10 seconds (Fig. 3). Put your ear close to chest and listen for heartbeat. *If no pulse or heartbeat . . .*

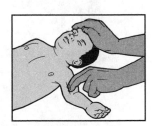
Figure 2

7. Phone EMS for Help
- Send someone to call.

OVER

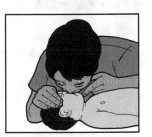
Figure 3

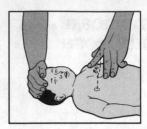

Figure 4

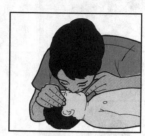

Figure 5

8. Position Your Hands

- Keep head tilted with one hand.
- Place index finger on breastbone, just below nipple level.
- Place next 2 fingers next to index finger, farther down breastbone. Lift index finger (Fig. 4). Use 2 middle fingers for next step.

9. Give 5 Compressions

- Bend your elbow.
- Use 2 fingers to depress breastbone ½ to 1 inch. Push straight down.
- Give 5 compressions in about 3 seconds.

10. Give 1 Slow Breath

- Seal your lips tightly around nose and mouth and give 1 breath (Fig. 5).
- Check pulse.
  If no pulse . . .

11. Repeat Cycles of 1 Breath and 5 Compressions for 10 Cycles

- Continue until baby revives or help arrives.

EMS or emergency phone number_____

EXTERNAL BLEEDING

1. Call EMS if Bleeding Is Severe

2. Wash Your Hands

- Wash hands. Put on sterile gloves if you have them.
- Remove loose debris from wound.

3. Apply Direct Pressure

- Put a barrier — layers of sterile dressings, clean cloth, or plastic wrap — between you and wound.
- Press dressing firmly (Fig. 1).
- Don't remove dressing. Put new dressings over soaked dressings. Keep pressing.

4. Elevate

- If no broken bone, raise wound above heart level.
  If person is still bleeding after 15 minutes . . .

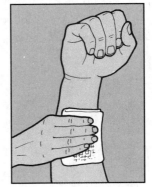

Figure 1

5. Apply Pressure Point Bleeding Control

- Use only when necessary, on arm or leg.
- Find pressure point (feel for pulse) and press artery against the bone (Fig. 2).
- Continue direct pressure and elevation.

6. Prevent Shock

- Lay victim flat. Raise feet. Cover with blanket.

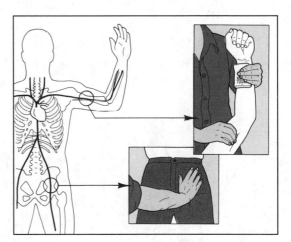

Figure 2

EMS or emergency phone number_____

Resources

Acquired Immunodeficiency Syndrome (AIDS)

AIDS Information Hotline
Public Health Service
(800) 342-AIDS
(800) 243-7889; Deaf and hearing impaired (TTY)
(800) 344-7432; Spanish-speaking
Provides information to the public on the prevention and spread of AIDS.

American Red Cross
Provides information on the prevention and spread of AIDS. Call your Red Cross chapter.

Alcoholism

Al-Anon and Alateen
(800) 356-9996
Provides printed materials on alcoholism specifically aimed at helping families.

Alcoholism and Drug Addiction Treatment Center
(800) 382-4357
Refers adolescents and adults to local facilities for help.

National Council on Alcoholism and Drug Dependence
(Hope)line
(800) NCA-CALL
Refers to local affiliates and provides written information on alcoholism and teenage drinking problems.

National Clearinghouse for Alcohol and Drug Information
(800) 729-6688
Information and publications on alcohol and other drugs.

Child Abuse

National Child Help Hotline
Child Help International Order of Foresters
(800) 422-4453
Provides counseling, referral, and reporting services concerning child abuse.

Parents Anonymous Hotline
(800) 421-0353
(800) 352-0386 in California
Provides information on and referrals for self-help groups for parents involved in child abuse.

Diabetes

American Diabetes Association
(800) 232-3472
(703) 549-1500 in Virginia and the District of Columbia metropolitan area
Provides free literature, newsletters, and information on diabetes health education and support group assistance.

Juvenile Diabetes Foundation International Hotline
(800) 223-1138
(212) 889-7575 in New York
Answers questions and provides brochures on juvenile diabetes. Gives referrals to physicians and clinics.

Drug Abuse

"Just Say No" Kids Club
(800) 258-2766
Responds to questions on how to start a club for 7- to 14-year-olds.

National Cocaine Hotline
(800) COCAINE
Answers questions on the health risks of cocaine for cocaine users and their friends and families. Provides referrals for counseling. A service of the Psychiatric Institute of America.

National Institute on Drug Abuse Helpline
(800) 662-HELP
Provides general information on drug abuse and on AIDS as it

relates to intravenous drug users. Also offers referrals.

National Clearinghouse for Alcohol
and Drug Information
(800) 729-6686
(301) 468-2600 in Maryland
Offers information and technical assistance to schools, parent groups, business and industry, and national organizations in developing drug abuse prevention activities. Does not provide crisis counseling, intervention, treatment, referral, or information on the pharmacology or criminal aspects of drugs.

Fitness

Women's Sports Foundation
(800) 227-3988
(212) 972-9170 in Alaska, Hawaii,
and New York City metropolitan
area
Provides information on women's sports, physical fitness, and sports medicine.

Hazardous Materials (Toxic Waste)

Household Products Disposal
Council
(202) 659-5535
Provides information and referrals on the proper disposal of household products.

Heart Disease

Heartline
(804) 965-6464
Answers questions and provides free literature on heart, health, cardiovascular diseases, and strokes. A service of the American Heart Association.

Lung Disease

Lung Line
National Asthma Center
(800) 222-5864
(303) 355-LUNG in Denver
Answers questions about asthma, emphysema, chronic bronchitis, allergies, juvenile rheumatoid arthritis, smoking, and other respiratory and immune system disorders. Callers' questions are answered by registered nurses. A service of the National Jewish Center for Immunology and Respiratory Medicine.

Mental Health

American Mental Health Fund
(800) 433-5959
(800) 826-2336 in Illinois
Makes available via recorded message the AMHF pamphlet that includes general information about the organization, mental health, and warning signs of mental illness.

Pesticides

National Pesticide
Telecommunications Network
Hotline
(800) 858-PEST
(806) 743-3091 in Texas
Responds to nonemergency questions concerning the effects, toxicology and symptoms, environmental effects, waste disposal and cleanup, and safe use of pesticides. A service of the Environmental Protection Agency and Texas Tech University.

Pregnancy

ASPO/Lamaze (American Society
for Psychoprophylaxis·in
Obstetrics)
(800) 368-4404
Provides list of local certified childbirth educators for people who are interested in the Lamaze birth method.

Safety

Consumer Product Safety
Commission
(800) 638-CPSC
Answers questions and provides materials on consumer product safety, including product hazards, product defects, and injuries sustained while using products. Covers only products used in and around the home, excluding automobiles, foods, drugs, cosmetics, boats, firearms, and pesticides.

Auto Safety Hotline
National Highway Traffic Safety
Administration
(800) 424-9393
(202) 366-0123 in the District of
Columbia
Provides information and referrals on the effectiveness of occupant protection devices, such as safety belts and child safety seats. Also gives information on auto recalls, auto-crash test results, tire quality reports, and other auto safety topics. Staffed by experts who investigate consumer complaints and provide assistance to resolve problems. Reports safety defects and gives referrals to other government agencies for consumer questions on warranties, service, and auto safety regulations.

National Safety Council
(800) 621-7619 for placing orders
(312) 527-4800 in Illinois
Provides posters, brochures, and booklets on safety and the prevention of accidents.

National Fire Protection Association
(800) 344-3555

Provides literature on fire safety and fire codes and standards.

Sudden Infant Death Syndrome

National SIDS Foundation
(800) 221-SIDS
(410) 964-8000

Provides literature and referrals on SIDS as well as information on support groups.

Trauma

American Trauma Society (ATS)
(800) 556-7890

Offers information to health professionals and the public on ATS activities. Answers questions about trauma and medical emergencies. Provides educational materials on how to reduce injuries.

Index

ABCs, 16, 17, 18, 19
  checking, 89
  See also Airway, protection;
    Breathing; Circulation
Abdominal cramps/pain as symptom:
  allergic reaction, 45
  chemical exposure or poison, 97,
    164
  head injury, 151
  internal bleeding, 62
  seizure, 168
  spinal injury, 176
  toxic reaction to bites or stings, 51
Abdominal pain. *See* Bleeding
Abdominal thrusts (Heimlich maneu-
    ver). *See* Choking
Abrasions (scrapes). *See* Wounds
Acetaminophen, 170
Agitation as drug overdose or with-
    drawal symptom, 126, 127
"A I D," 13–14. *See also* Harming vic-
    tim; Help, calling for
AIDS (acquired immunodeficiency syn-
    drome), transmission of, 25–
    26.
  See also Disease transmission
"Air ambulances," 32
Air-borne diseases. *See* Disease trans-
    mission
Airway, obstructed. *See* Choking; Facial
    Injury
Airway, protection of, 14, 16
  opening of, 17
  recovery position and, 20
  vomiting and, 65, 151

  See also Breathing Problems
Airway burns. *See* Burns
Airway or chest injury. *See* Breathing
    Problems
Alcohol, avoidance of:
  when driving, 280
  in head injury, 150
  in heat illness, 155, 157
  in hypothermia, 120
  with medications, 220
  and nosebleed, 163
  and swimming, 275
Alcohol abuse. *See* Drug Abuse
Alertness, decreasing:
  as symptom of head injury, 144,
    148
  as symptom of shock:
    bites and stings, 51
    bleeding, 62
    burns, 85
    spinal injury, 176
  See also Confused or irrational be-
    havior as symptom; Drowsiness
    as symptom
Allergic Reaction, 45–47
  from bite or sting, 50, 51, 52
  from chemical exposure, 97, 99
  delayed, 50, 51
  first aid for, 46–47
  hives as, 45, 51, 97
  mild to moderate (anaphylactic), 45,
    46
  severe (anaphylaxis), 45, 47
    and anaphylactic shock, 45
  and shock, 172, 173

  signs and symptoms, 45
Ambulance, transportation by, 31–32,
  35
American Red Cross:
  courses offered by, 5, 16,
  founding of, 240
Amphetamines, effect of. *See* Drug
  Abuse
Amputation, 48–49
  first aid for, 48–49
  how to save amputated part, 48, 49,
    130
  signs and symptoms, 48
Anaphylaxis. *See* Allergic Reaction
Angina. *See* Heart Attack
Animals:
  bites from, *see* Bites and Stings
  safety around, 260–261
Ankle injury. *See* Bone, Joint, and Mus-
    cle Injuries
Antivenins. *See* Bites and Stings
Anxiety as symptom:
  drug withdrawal, 127
  heart attack, 153
  shock, 173
Appetite loss as symptom of poisoning,
  164
Arm injury. *See* Bone, Joint, and Mus-
    cle Injuries
Arrest, cardiopulmonary. *See* Cardio-
    pulmonary Arrest
Arrest, respiratory. *See* Cardiopulmo-
    nary Arrest
Arrival at scene of emergency. *See*
  Emergency

309

Choking *(cont.)*
  facial injury and, 144
  first aid for, 109–117
  gagging, 108
  in infant:
    conscious, 114–115
    unconscious, 115–117
  in large or pregnant victim, 112–113
  seizure associated with, 111, 169
  signs and symptoms, 108
  See also Airway, protection or clearing of
Circulation, 15
  checking, 17, 18, 19
  poor, and hypothermia, 118
  See also Pulse
Closets. *See* Storage areas, safety of
Clothes drag technique. *See* Moving the victim
Cocaine, effects of. *See* Drug Abuse
Cold Exposure, 117–120
  in drowning, 121, 122
  first aid for, 118–120
  frostbite, 117, 118–119
  hypothermia, 117, 118, 119–120, 122, 173
  and shock, 173
  signs and symptoms, 118
Collarbone injury. *See* Bone, Joint, and Muscle Injuries
Colorado tick fever, 52
Communication with victim, guidelines for, 22
Concussion. *See* Head Injury
Cone shell, 61. *See also* Bites and Stings
Confused or irrational behavior as symptom, 22
  and consent of victim, 4
  and decision making by victim, 14
  drug overdose or withdrawal, 126, 127
  emotional trauma, 24
  head injury, 144, 148, 149, 151
  heat illness, 156, 157
  hyperglycemia, 184
  hypoglycemia, 185
  hypothermia, 118
  seizure, 169
  shock, 173
Consciousness, checking for, 16. *See also* Unconsciousness; Unconsciousness as symptom or reaction

Consent of victim, 4–5, 14, 15
  hospital consent form, 35
  implied, 4
Contact lenses, 137, 138, 141
  how to remove, 140
  See also Eye Injury
Convulsions. *See* Seizures
Cough as symptom:
  airway burn, 85
  breathing problem, 80, 110
  poisoning, 165
  See also Choking
CPR. *See* Cardiopulmonary Arrest
Cramp, muscle. *See* Bone, Joint, and Muscle Injuries
Cramps. *See* Heat Illnesses
Cramps, abdominal. *See* Abdominal cramps/pain as symptom
Crime. *See* Victims of crime
Croup. *See* Breathing Problems
Cuts and tears (lacerations). *See* Wounds

Death of victim, 24
Dehydration:
  avoidance of, in strenuous activity, 266
  and heat illness, 155, 157
  of infant, 170
  as symptom of injury or illness, 151, 170
  See also Thirst, extreme, as symptom
Delivery, of child. *See* Childbirth
Dental injuries. *See* Facial Injury
Depressants, effect of. *See* Drug Abuse
Depression as symptom:
  drug withdrawal, 127
  poisoning, 164
Diabetes:
  and eye problems, 136
  and frostbite, 118
  and heart attack, 153
  and seizures, 169
  and wounds, 187
Diabetic reaction. *See* Unconsciousness
Diarrhea as symptom:
  in infant, 151
  in poisoning, 164
  of shock, 173
Difficulty breathing. *See* Breathing Problems
Disaster survival, 240–255
  accident involving hazardous materials, 252–255

earthquakes, 242, 243, 251, 285
floods, 242, 249–250, 284
guidelines for, 247
hurricanes, 242, 250–251, 284
planning for, 241–246
  evacuation plans, 243–246
  sheltering in place, 255
technological disasters, 242, 252–255
thunderstorms, 242, 247–249, 285
  and danger from lightning, 234, 247–248
tornadoes, 242, 249, 284
See also Fire prevention, preparedness, and survival
Discharge from injured area, 52. *See also* Infection, signs of
Disease transmission:
  AIDS, 25–26
  air-borne, 26
  blood-borne, 25–26
  in childbirth, precautions against, 101
  hepatitis, 25
  prevention of, 25–26, 101
Dislocations. *See* Bone, Joint, and Muscle Injuries
Disorientation. *See* Confused or irrational behavior as symptom
Dizziness. *See* Unconsciousness
Dizziness/weakness as symptom:
  allergic reaction, 45, 51
  bite or sting, 50, 51
  bleeding, 62
  chemical exposure, 97, 164
  ear injury, 130
  head injury, 149
  heart attack, 153
  heat illness, 155, 156
  hyperventilation, 81
  hypothermia, 118
  poisoning, 164, 165
  shock, 173
  spinal injury, 176
  stroke, 181
Double vision. *See* Vision, double or impaired, as symptom
DPT vaccination, 188
Dressings, applying, 191
Dressings for first aid kit, 6
Drooling:
  as symptom of croup, 83
  as symptom of seizure, 169
  of unconscious victim, 174

312   **Index**

Seizures (*cont.*)
  illnesses or injuries associated with, 169
  in poisoning, 165, 168, 169
  signs and symptoms, 169
Sensation, loss of, as symptom:
  spinal injury, 176
  wound, 188
  See also Numbness or tingling as symptom
Septic shock. *See* Shock
Sexual abuse. *See* Genital Injury
Sheltering in place, 255
Shock, 172–174
  allergic reaction and, 47, 51, 172, 173
  amputation and, 49
  bites and stings and, 55, 58, 60
  bleeding and, 64, 65
  burns and, 86, 87, 88
  first aid for:
    with no spinal injury, 173–174
    with spinal injury, 174
  insulin, 184
  septic, 173
  signs and symptoms, 173
  and vomiting or drooling, 174
Shock, anaphylactic. *See* Allergic Reaction
Shock, electrical. *See* Electrical Injury
Shock as symptom:
  bleeding, 62
  burn, 85
  with fever, serious problem, 170
  heart attack, 153
  spinal injury, 176
Shoulder injury. *See* Bone, Joint, and Muscle Injuries (arm)
Skin color and temperature. *See* Flushed face as symptom; Lips; Pale, clammy, or bluish skin as symptom; Redness; Temperature, body
Skin rash as symptom:
  with fever, serious problem, 170
  poisoning, 165
Skull, injuries to. *See* Head Injury
Sleepiness. *See* Drowsiness as symptom
Slings. *See* Splints and slings
Slurred speech. *See* Speech, slurred or loss of, as symptom
Smoke detectors, 235–236

Smoking:
  and guidelines for fire prevention, 231–232
  and hypothermia, 118, 120
Snakebites, nonvenomous. *See* Wounds, puncture, 195
Snakebites, venomous. *See* Bites and Stings
Snakes:
  poisonous, in North America, 56, 262
  safety around, 261–262
Snorting as symptom of seizure, 169
Speech, slurred or loss of, as symptom:
  alcohol abuse, 126
  bite or sting, 50
  head injury, 149
  hypothermia, 118
  poisoning, 165
  stroke, 181
  TIA (transient ischemic attack), 181
Spider bites, venomous. *See* Bites and Stings
Spinal Injury, 175–180
  checking for, 17
  first aid for, 176–180
  and head tilt/chin lift, 17, 89
  moving the victim of, 18, 20–21, 174, 176, 177, 178–179, 180
  and shock, 173, 174, 176
  signs and symptoms, 176
  and vomiting, 177
Splinters. *See* Wounds
Splints and slings, 73–78
  how to apply, 74–76
  See also Bandage(s); Moving the victim
Sports injuries. *See* Bone, Joint, and Muscle Injuries
Sports safety, 267–270
  how to prevent injuries, 267–269
  in children, 269–270
  See also Water safety
Sprains. *See* Bone, Joint, and Muscle Injuries
Stairs, safety of. *See* Living room/stairs, safety of
Stiff jaw (lockjaw) as tetanus symptom, 188
Stiff muscles: hypothermia and, 118.
  See also Bone, Joint, and Muscle Injuries
Stiff neck as symptom:
  with fever, serious problem, 170
  head injury, 149, 151

Stimulants, effect of. *See* Drug Abuse
Stings. *See* Bites and Stings
Stool, blood in, 62. *See also* Bleeding
Storage areas, safety of, 226
  child-proofing for, 227
  general precautions, 227
Storm watch and warning, difference between, 241
Strains. *See* Bone, Joint, and Muscle Injuries
Stroke, 181–182
  drug overdose as cause of, 126, 127
  first aid for, 181–182
  heart attack and, 152
  signs and symptoms, 181
Stupor as symptom of poisoning, 165
Substance abuse. *See* Drug Abuse
Sunstroke (heatstroke). *See* Heat Illnesses
Survival in disaster. *See* Disaster survival
"Survival pack" for hiking, 265
Swallowing, difficulty in, as symptom:
  allergic reaction, 45, 51
  chemical exposure, 97, 164
  poisoning, 164, 165
Swallowing poison (ingestion). *See* Poison
Sweating as symptom:
  bite or sting, 50
  drug overdose or withdrawal, 126, 127
  heart attack, 153
  heat illness, 155
  hypoglycemia, 185
Swelling of eyes, face, or tongue as symptom:
  allergic reaction, 45, 51
  chemical exposure, 97
Swelling of injured area:
  after application of splint, 76
  as sign of ear injury, 130
  as sign of infection, 52, 86, 189
  as sign of bone, joint, or muscle injury, 70
  as sign of genital injury, 146
  in zipper injury, 198
Swimming:
  in ocean, 279
  in pools, 277–278
  in ponds, lakes, or rivers, 278–279
  See also Drowning
Swollen lymph nodes, as sign of infection, 52
Synovial fluid, synovium, 69, 70

318   **Index**

Teeth, loose, broken, or missing. *See* Facial Injury

Telephone numbers, emergency, 5, 30–31, 33

Temperature, body:
  and febrile seizures, 168–169, 170
  and fever as reaction to or symptom of:
    bites or stings, 51, 52
    croup, 83
    drug abuse, 127
    poisoning, 164
    with skin rash, serious problem, 170
  heat illness and, 156–159
  See also Pale, clammy, or bluish skin as symptom

Tendon, 69

Tendon, severed. *See* Bone, Joint, and Muscle Injuries

Tendonitis. *See* Bone, Joint, and Muscle Injuries

Tetanus, 188
  from bite or sting, 50, 261

Tetanus immunizations:
  for bites and stings, 52
  for burns, 85, 87
  effectiveness of, 188
  for facial injury, 144
  for wounds, 65, 188

Thirst, extreme, as symptom:
  heat exhaustion, 156
  hyperglycemia, 184
  shock, 173
  See also Dehydration

Three-person hammock carry. *See* Moving the victim

Thunderstorms. *See* Disaster survival

TIA (Transient ischemic attack), 181. *See also* Stroke

Tick bites, 52–53. *See also* Bites and Stings

Tingling. *See* Numbness or tingling as symptom

Toe injury. *See* Bone, Joint, and Muscle Injuries; Burns; Cold Exposure (frostbite)

Tooth injury. *See also* Facial Injury

Tornadoes. *See* Disaster survival

Toxic reaction:
  to bites or stings, 51
  to chemical exposure, 98–99
  diabetic, 184–185

Transient ischemic attack (TIA), 181.

See also Stroke

Transmission of illness. *See* Disease transmission

Transportation (of victim):
  by air, 32
  by ambulance, 31–32, 35
  by rescuer, 35
  See also Moving the victim

Tremors as symptom of drug abuse or withdrawal, 127

Two-handed seat carry. *See* Moving the victim

Unconsciousness, 182–186
  checking for consciousness, 16
  and clues to what happened, 11, 165
  fainting, 183
    hyperventilation and, 84
  first aid for, 14–18, 182–186
    in breathing problems, 83
    in choking, 110–111, 112–113, 115–117
    in diabetic emergency, 185
    in drowning, 124
    in head injury, 149–150
    in heart attack, 154–155
    in infant, 95–96, 115–117
    in shock, 173–174
  and implied consent, 4
  insulin (diabetic) reaction, 184–185
  and recovery position, 183
    when to use, 20, 81, 124, 128, 143, 151, 171
  and rescuer as advocate, 36
  signs and symptoms, 182
  See also Unconsciousness as symptom or reaction

Unconsciousness as symptom or reaction:
  allergy, 45, 47
  bites or stings, 51
  cardiopulmonary arrest, 90
  chemical exposure, 97, 98
  choking, 108
  drug overdose, 126
  electrical injury, 132
  head injury, 148, 150
  heart attack, 153
  heat illnesses, 156, 157
  hypothermia, 118
  poisoning, 165
  seizure, 169
  shock, 173

spinal injury, 176

stroke, 181

See also Alertness, decreasing

Underwriters Laboratory (UL), 216, 237

"Urgent care center," 32. *See also* Emergency facilities

Urination, frequent, as symptom of hyperglycemia, 184. *See also* Bladder control, loss of, as symptom

Urine:
  dark colored, heatstroke and, 156
  leakage in genital injury, 146

Urine, blood in. *See* Bleeding

Vagina, bleeding from, 62. *See also* Bleeding; Genital Injury

Venomous bites and stings. *See* Bites and Stings

Victims of crime, 23–24

Viruses, transmission of, 25–26
  See also Disease transmission

Vision, double or impaired, as symptom:
  alcohol abuse, 126
  eye injury, 136
  head injury, 144, 149
  poisoning, 165
  stroke, 181

Vomit, blood in. *See* Bleeding

Vomiting. *See* Head Injury; Nausea or vomiting as symptom; Poison

Watch and warning, storm, difference between, 241

Water safety, 274–279
  See also Drowning

Weakness. *See* Dizziness/weakness as symptom

Weather. *See* Auto safety; Disaster survival

Wheezing. *See* Breathing Problems

Wilderness rescue, 266–267

Withdrawal, drug or alcohol. *See* Drug Abuse

Wounds, 186–198
  chest ("sucking"), 82–83
  cuts and tears (lacerations), 194–195
  with embedded object, 63, 82, 148, 196, 197–198
  first aid for, 189–198
  fishhook removal, 197–198
  how to bandage, 190–193
  puncture, 195–196 (*see also* Bites and Stings)

American Red Cross Courses and Programs

For information on Red Cross courses and programs, contact your local Red Cross chapter. Red Cross health and safety courses and programs include:

- American Red Cross Community CPR
- American Red Cross Adult CPR
- American Red Cross CPR: Infant and Child
- American Red Cross Basic Aid Training (BAT) (for children)
- American Red Cross Learn to Swim Courses
- American Red Cross Longfellow's Whale Tales (for children)
- American Red Cross Infant and Preschool Aquatic Program

- American Red Cross Standard First Aid
- American Red Cross First Aid: Responding to Emergencies
- American Red Cross Basic Water Safety
- American Red Cross Emergency Water Safety
- American Red Cross Safety Training for Swim Coaches
- American Red Cross Basic Lifeguarding
- American Red Cross Lifeguard Training
- American Red Cross Basic Sailing

- American Red Cross Canoeing
- American Red Cross Kayaking
- American Red Cross Child Care Course
- American Red Cross Reaching Adolescents and Parents (RAP)
- American Red Cross Hispanic HIV/AIDS Program
- American Red Cross African American HIV/AIDS Program
- American Red Cross Workplace HIV/AIDS Program

Not all courses are available from all Red Cross units.